ALLOW GOD
TO WEAR YOUR FACE

SPIRITUAL CARE FOR THOSE WHO ARE ILL

Alice G. Knotts, M.Div., Ph. D.

Other books by this author:

Lifting Up Hope, Living Out Justice:
Methodist Women and the Social Gospel
2007

Selected for the United Methodist Women's 2009 Reading Program,
Women's Division, General Board of Global Ministries

∞

Fellowship of Love:
Methodist Women Changing
American Racial Attitudes, 1920-1968
1996
Winner of the Jesse Lee Prize in United Methodist history.

∞

To Transform the World:
Vital United Methodist Campus Ministries 2009
Edited by this author
For this work Knotts received the
Don Shockley Award for Contribution to Intellectual Life.

PRAISE FOR *ALLOW GOD TO WEAR YOUR FACE*

If you visit people who are sick, you need this book. Alice Knotts provides a theologically grounded guide to being supportive, pastoral and useful to those who are sick and to their families. What do you say to a terminal patient, to a parent who has lost a child, to a beaten spouse or a church member facing surgery? Alice has you in mind. *Allow God to Wear Your Face* provides practical and spiritually rich guidance. You will buy this book and pass it along to all those you know who care for others.

Ann Craig
former Executive Secretary for Spiritual and Theological Development
Women's Division, General Board of Global Ministries
The United Methodist Church

When people are sick, especially when experiencing serious illness, they face unique challenges and opportunities. Even though we may mean well, it can feel like what we say to them is inadequate; hollow platitudes or helpless bromides. The author of *Allow God to Wear Your Face* shares from her extensive and intensive experiences as a chaplain and pastor to encourage the sacred art of listening. She describes how caregivers can come alongside and walk with those who are sick instead of preaching or giving advice. Her practical wisdom, when followed, can help prevent embarrassing pitfalls while facilitating the healing of relationships, emotions, spirit and even the body.

Chaplain Ray Mitchell
Director of Spiritual Care and Patient Advocacy
Yuma Regional Medical Center

Alice Knotts has written a perceptive and sensitive book which reflects the combination of her scholarship and experience. The book is thoroughly practical and eminently useful for both lay and clergy persons who seek to care for the sick and dying and their families. It will be a valuable resource that those in this work of all Christians will reach for over and over.

The Rev. Dr. Gayle Carlton Felton
Duke Divinity School former faculty member
Authored Methodism's official documents on sacraments

Allow God to Wear Your Face is a practical guide for persons who want to make meaningful visits to relatives and friends who are sick. The goal of visits is to offer our self to others. Jesus provides the example of how to show God's love for those who are sick. Love becomes: Listen, Observe, Value and Engage. The book is well illustrated with examples of situations one may encounter when visiting. Practical resources are offered, including sample words of comfort and prayers. The book would be of great value to pastors, church visitors, Stephens Ministers, students in Clinical Pastoral Education and anyone who visits relatives or friends who are sick.

The Rev. Tom Carter, Chaplain
Director of Endorsement
General Board of Higher Education and Ministry
The United Methodist Church

The book is a practical guide to visiting ill persons for spiritual support from the Protestant Christian understanding of faith. Persons who are feeling called to minister to the sick but have not been trained will find the information very helpful in their preparation. The book provides a great resource for local congregations to use when equipping persons to become pastoral visitors.

The Rev. Sally A. Schwab, Chaplain
2010 President of the Association for Clinical Pastoral Education
Heartland Regional Medical Center, St. Joseph, Missouri

United Methodist Women, spiritual friends and other members of congregations invest themselves in building supporting community. When a member of the community or someone's family member becomes ill, we sometimes wonder about what is the best thing to do or say. This little book will help you to answer just this question and feel more confident as you express God's love in this way. This is one to read, save and read again.

Harriett Jane Olson, Deputy General Secretary
Women's Division, General Board of Global Ministries
The United Methodist Church

ALLOW GOD TO WEAR YOUR FACE

SPIRITUAL CARE FOR THOSE WHO ARE ILL

Alice G. Knotts, M.Div., Ph. D.

Frontrowlving Press
PO Box 19291
San Diego, CA 92159
619-955-0925
frontrowliving@yahoo.com

ISBN: 978-0-9794194-1-6

Book and cover design by Jaimie Knapp and Brenda Riddell.
The nautilus design represents balance and harmony.

Cover Photo: San Diego sunset © Alice G. Knotts

The Lord gives strength to those who are weary.
Even young people get tired, then stumble and fall.
But those who trust the Lord will find new strength.
They will be strong like eagles, soaring upward on wings;
they will walk and run without getting tired.

Isaiah 40:29-31
CEV

Allow God to Wear Your Face:
Spiritual Care for Those Who Are Ill

Quotations from scripture are from the Contemporary English Version of the Bible. *Holy Bible, Contemporary English Version* (New York, NY: American Bible Society, 1995).

To my daughter, Laura Patricia Knotts Bowman
And granddaughter, Ellie Grace Bowman

ACKNOWLEDGMENTS

I wish to thank people who helped with the preparation, editing, and reading of this book in its various stages of development. The invitation to write came from the Women's Division of the Board of the Board of Global Ministries of The United Methodist Church and was mentored by Ann Craig. Staff members of the Department of Spiritual Care and Patient Advocacy at Yuma Regional Medical Center and patients there provided me with training and experiences in the field of spiritual care.

In fulfilling my desire to provide wide access to ordinary people on the theme of how to do spiritual care, friends and colleagues helped with reading, editing, and suggestions to make this book helpful to you. I wish to thank The Rev. Alice Ann Glenn, Dr. Beth Cooper, Chaplain Dean Yamamoto, Dr. Gayle Felton, and Chaplain Ray Mitchell. I thank those who took the time to read the book and provide endorsements from their various perspectives as theologians, chaplains, pastors, directors of spiritual care, and endorsers of chaplains, as well as teachers of pastors and chaplains who provide spiritual care. I appreciate receiving endorsements from Dr. Gayle Felton and Chaplains Tom Carter, Sally Schwab, Harriett Jane Olson, Ann Craig and Ray Mitchell. Thanks go to Brenda Riddell and Jaimie Knapp for graphic design and John Coffey for assistance with publishing.

CONTENTS

SPIRITUAL CARE FOR THOSE WHO ARE ILL I

PRAISE FOR *ALLOW GOD TO WEAR YOUR FACE* IV

SPIRITUAL CARE FOR THOSE WHO ARE ILL VII

ACKNOWLEDGMENTS XI

PREFACE XV

PART I. BE A CENTERED SPIRITUAL CARE VISITOR 1

INTRODUCTION 3

ALLOW GOD TO WEAR YOUR FACE 4

LIFE'S CHALLENGES 5

CHRISTIAN TRADITION 6

DEFINING A SPIRITUAL CARE VISIT 9

GETTING OFF TO A QUICK START 9

PART II. SHOW L.O.V.E. 13

SPIRITUAL CARE SHOWS LOVE 15

LISTEN 15

OBSERVE 17

VALUE 18

ENGAGE 21

PART III. SPIRITUAL CARE TO FIT THE SITUATION 23

COMMON FACTORS IN SPIRITUAL CARE VISITS 25

THE BASICS OF SPIRITUAL CARE 26

"WHAT SHOULD I SAY AND DO?" QUIZ 26

FETAL DEMISE 29

DOMESTIC VIOLENCE 31

CHRONIC ILLNESS 31

TEEN AGE ACCIDENT 32

HEART PATIENT 33

CANCER 34

DYING 35

HIV/AIDS 36

DEMENTIA 37

DIABETES 39

SUDDEN DEATH 39

CATASTROPHE.. 42

CONCLUSION 43

PART IV. RESOURCES.. 45

ADVANCE DIRECTIVE.. 47

PATIENT ADVOCACY... 47

PRE-SURGERY... 48

POST-SURGERY 48

HOME CARE.. 48

HOSPICE 49

EXTENDED CARE FACILITY... 49

RELIGIOUS, ETHNIC AND CULTURAL SENSITIVITY................................ 49

ASSESSING SPIRITUAL CARE NEEDS... 50

ORGAN AND TISSUE DONATION.. 50

FAVORITE WORDS OF COMFORT FROM THE BIBLE 51

PRAYERS 52

LITURGIES 54

ANOINTING THE SICK.. 54

DEDICATION OF A CHILD WHO IS DYING OR WHO HAS DIED........... 54

BAPTISM FOR A CHILD 55

COMMUNION.. 56

HOSPICE RESOURCES 59

BOOKS AND RESOURCES... 60

PREFACE

This book provides an introduction and resources for persons who wish to provide spiritual care. It is addressed to people who want to help a sick friend; to laity, volunteers with Stephen Ministries, seminarians, local pastors and ordained persons; to health care workers, nurses and doctors; to people in hospitals or home settings; to church members and clinical pastoral education students. Spiritual care helps with healing.

While professional credentials are not required to provide spiritual care, wisdom is essential. This guide can help. You may first read this book for training or orientation purposes and then turn to it again and again for helpful guidance, prayers and resources.

Good spiritual care does not ask patients to change their religious preference but instead asks questions to guide those who are ill to do their own spiritual work. This guide offers Christian resources to providers of spiritual care. It does not impose a way of thinking on patients but helps caregivers know appropriate questions to ask.

Some of the resources are helpful for persons who have no medical background or no church background. Others, such as the sacraments of Holy Communion and Baptism, are for ordained ministers and for local pastors who have pastoral assignments and whose limited scope of sacramental responsibility is broadly defined as "people within or related to the community or ministry setting being served."

If you have never spent much time with the Bible, you may discover that people who have heard and read the Bible over many years are nurtured by the power of its texts and images, its stories, and the way it lifts people up and gives hope. The Bible is more than a text. It becomes lived experience in a faith community. Community is an important factor in healing.[1]

When you are part of a team offering health care, each person has responsibilities but it takes the whole team to provide quality care. Teams thrive on good communication and cooperation. This guide helps you know what to say and do.

Thank you for caring for those who are ill.

PART I

Be a Centered
Spiritual Care Visitor

INTRODUCTION

My first car was a small gray Volvo shaped almost like a Volkswagen bug. It was part of a miracle package. I set out from Oregon and went to New Jersey to start life after graduate school. I asked friends for a place to stay temporarily. In one week I looked for work, landed a job, found a place to live, and bought the old Volvo for $500. Through this experience I felt that God was looking out for me during a time of transition and risk. Later, when I felt scared or intimidated, not knowing how I was going to get through a tough situation, I would recall this time and remind myself that I could do hard things with God's help.

While it is possible to break down my miracle week into lots of pieces of a puzzle and put it back together without ever mentioning God, I never wanted to do that. All the component pieces were part of a spiritual life cultivated over time—the habits of making friends, attending church, living frugally, saving money, praying, trusting God, listening for God's call in my life, and responding with a willing "Yes!"

Spiritual habits cultivated over time are needed in a time of sickness and crisis. When you are a spiritual care visitor, one of your tasks is to help patients draw from their well of spiritual resources to assist with their healing. This book will help you know how to listen to the patient and discern what spiritual resources and gifts they have already cultivated and internalized.

Where do sick people get nourishment for their soul? Nourishment comes from God. Precisely when they are worried, don't know the outcome, have pain, and are feeling terrible, faith is tested. Life's big questions hit. Why did this happen? Will I get well? What if I die? Faith means trusting God when you don't know what will happen to you. It means connecting to the inner resources that God provides.

The practice of Christian living cultivates daily habits that help people deal with emergencies. To prepare for an earthquake you might set aside flashlights, jackets, food and water. Part of the task of a spiritual care visitor is to help people do the soul work that helps them survive hard times. You can help people cultivate the habits of Christian living so that the resources of a relationship with God are there to draw on in times of need.

This book is a simple guide for persons who wish to make their visits with sick people more meaningful and effective. When you visit someone who is sick, you are part of a healing team. Doctors, nurses, family, friends, church, synagogue and mosque can work together to put support around someone who is sick. It's awesome when people on the healing team bring a maximum amount of support.

When you, the spiritual caregiver, know what you are doing, have confidence, skills and resources at your fingertips, your visit can make a perceptible difference. You might not see the results right away, but sometimes you do. It is very rewarding.

Jesus showed us that there is more to healing than science can explain. Emotional issues, psychological issues, stress, worries, depression, grief, fear, trauma, abuse, addiction, guilt, and shame affect all of us, our bodies and our health. Dr. Joan Guntzelman says, "Nobody gets over anything" because everything that we experience is incorporated into who we are. All too often we carry around a load of un-grieved loss. Even though bad things happen to everyone, sometimes we let them get us down. A bad attitude makes us feel worse. Nobody gives us our attitude. We choose it. A good attitude helps us get better.

ALLOW GOD TO WEAR YOUR FACE

You will be, or are already, spending time with sick people. As a spiritual caregiver you can be helpful even if you are not an expert in medicine, nursing, psychology or addiction. The greatest gift that you have to offer is your calm, spiritual, non-anxious presence. When you visit, you become a channel for God's presence. The sick person is at the center, receiving love and care. You take an assisting role. With your presence, you provide an opportunity for sick persons to feel closer to God, to feel as though God loves them and sustains them through a difficult time, and to feel that they are accepted and appreciated. Not everyone will experience this with you. Your task is to provide the setting and create the opportunity.

You may be surprised when a patient says and does something that helps heal you. When you bring your whole self into the setting and are authentic, you are aware that in life you are also a patient. You, too, are wounded. You enter the presence of a sick person as one who knows what it means to hurt, but you focus on the patient. When that happens, you are additionally blessed as you feel God working through a patient to mend your life. Sometimes the patients are aware of feeling their power and healing capacity.

The best gift we have to offer is our self and our respect for the other person. We need self-awareness and the ability to use the present moment. We need to be our true self. Author John Donne said, "God is present in you as you."

Suffering is a frequent entry point to the sacred. It helps us become spiritually aware. Your listening can help people let go of troubles. Out of grieving comes renewal. Illness, aging and death are precious times of transition and learning. You, the visitor, help open up this treasure. It's rewarding. Many people, even children, have a sense of the sacred. A point of sickness is a time when God enters the room and is embodied in us. Patients may see or feel Jesus or God with them. Allow God to wear your face.

LIFE'S CHALLENGES

Spiritual growth emerges out of life's challenges. Life is a journey of facing challenges, overcoming setbacks, and finding our potential. We get trapped in our habits. Healing is more than healing our body. It is emotional as well as physical. Illness can be a time when we stop to reflect about our life. We have a special opportunity for self-renewal or transformation. We may suddenly become aware of something new. There's more room for God to work when we pay attention and are aware. Illness is an opportunity to break habitual ways of doing things and create new awareness, new thoughts and new ways of relating.[2] We powerfully shape life with our thoughts, values, attitudes, and feelings, either living them out or choosing our path.

Self-consciousness of these aspects of life makes it possible for us to birth new choices. "Repent" means "turn around," but it also can mean "you can go beyond where you are." Jesus told his disciples, "I've been with you and you still don't see." Spirituality means waking up, awakening. In awareness is healing, salvation, spirituality and love. To be born and reborn we have to let go and let part of ourselves die—attitudes, expectations, hopes, dreams, and abilities. This is the way life is. We have seasons. We have losses. Christians believe that unless these die, we don't get life. The groundwork for new life is death. You bury a seed to grow something new.

CHRISTIAN TRADITION

When it came to helping sick people, Jesus frequently got into trouble for doing the wrong thing. Jesus' critics, the Pharisees, chewed him out for healing on the Sabbath, offering forgiveness, and helping people who didn't deserve it. Jesus didn't always follow the religious customs of his day because he saw what could happen. Sometimes the social customs and rules stunted people's lives and spirits. That's why Jesus crossed social boundaries. He seemed to know that people's emotions, fears, guilt and shame could have physical symptoms. Jesus assumed that he could be a channel of God's forgiveness. God's forgiveness heals.

Of the four gospel writers, Luke was most interested in Jesus' healing ministry. Luke 13:10-17 tells a story about a day when Jesus was outside the synagogue in a small town. He healed a woman who had been bent over for eighteen years and could not straighten up. The man in charge of the synagogue was angry with Jesus for healing on the Sabbath. Healing hurting people was so important to Jesus that he was willing to break the Sabbath custom to do it. Luke reported, "Everyone in the crowd was happy about the wonderful things [Jesus] was doing."

Jesus believed that by helping people with their need he showed God's love for them. Sometimes Jesus could see past what people asked for to a deeper need. More than once Jesus asked people what they needed.

Luke wrote about a time when Jesus and his disciples were walking to Jericho. By this time Jesus was well known for healing people, and crowds of people were following him. A blind man who sat begging beside the road heard the crowd and asked what was happening. When he heard that it was Jesus, he called out. Jesus' followers told the blind man to be quiet, but he called out even louder. Jesus stopped and asked, "What do you want me to do for you?" Luke 18:41-43.

Jesus' question is an appropriate one. When someone is sick, it doesn't matter if you can ride a unicycle and juggle or what your talents are. You do not go to entertain a patient, but rather to be present and focused on the patient's need.

The blind man responded to Jesus saying, "Lord, I want to see!" Jesus replied, "Look and you will see! Your eyes are healed because of your faith." Luke tells us that right away the blind man could see. He went with Jesus and started thanking God. When the crowds saw what happened they praised God.

While we don't know all the circumstances of the blind man's healing, we do know several things.

1. Good spiritual care can facilitate healing. Spiritual care provided by a faith community and nurtured in the life of a person of faith can help people deal with illness and death. Faith sustains.
2. When people reach beyond their own resources to ask God to help them, they open up channels for healing that are not available if they simply aim to heal by themselves.
3. Attitudes make a big difference in healing. People who thank God and who express gratitude for incremental steps in the healing process have a helpful attitude.
4. Health is related to our emotions. When people replace fear with trust and let go of anger, they are doing spiritual work. When we surround ill persons with prayer, and when ill ones feel safe, loved, forgiven, nurtured and cared for, they do better emotionally.

If Jesus had wanted to keep his hands clean, he wouldn't have taken his ministry into the roads of Galilee and the streets of Jerusalem. One day, when Jesus was in the middle of a crowd of people on his way to heal a girl, he felt power drain away. An unnamed woman who sought to be healed touched the hem of his cloak, believing that coming this close to Jesus she would be healed. (Luke 8:42b-48) The woman had been spotting and bleeding for twelve years. In all that time, she was unable to meet the requirements of Jewish law to become ritually clean. Her touch was enough to make Jesus unclean under Jewish customs.

Jesus did not turn to ask, "Why did you do that?" Instead, he saw the woman and her need. He listened while she told him her life story. This was part of her healing, too. The result was that a person who had spent most of her life being isolated from other people, rejected by them because of her condition, was given a fresh opportunity to be integrated into the community.

Notice two important themes. In visiting the sick, occasionally you will meet people who are socially isolated and whose illnesses keep them even further apart from others. Like Jesus, you may be part of the healing process that helps isolated people become part of a community again. Notice a pattern in biblical stories.[3] Where two or more are gathered in Jesus' name, the power of God's love is at work. You come representing this power.

When the early Christian church described the gifts of its leaders for ministry and parceled out the tasks of ministry, it listed healing the sick along with teaching, preaching, administration and caring for the needy. (Acts 2:43-45, 9:32-41; I Cor. 12:27-28, 30) You are embarking on one of the oldest forms of Christian ministry that is part of the ministry of all Christians. The United Methodist Book of Discipline declares:

Ministry in the Christian church is derived from the ministry of Christ, who calls all persons to receive God's gift of salvation and follow in the way of love and service. The whole church receives and accepts this call, and all Christians participate in this continuing ministry.[4]

In the 1730s in England, John Wesley guided a group of students at Oxford University known as the Holy Club. Wesley was engaged in a search for his own salvation. He established habits for living a heavily scheduled life that included visiting people who were sick or in prison and praying for them. He practiced an age-old discipline of Christian living in which reaching out to others was important as are reading the Bible and taking Holy Communion. Later, as he became pastor to coal miners, their families and poor people from small towns all over the countryside, he wrote a book that gave people access to medical remedies, herbal and otherwise, that were accessible and inexpensive. He tried the remedies himself and commented on their effectiveness! He opened free clinics in London and Bristol to serve poor people. Later, churches in the Americas opened hospitals.

Women's organizations from various emerging Christian branches have long encouraged women to visit the sick. Since 1884, Methodist women trained as deaconesses became professional laywomen (certified, not ordained) who undertook ministries of service. They started many hospitals. Currently, women from many churches provide resources, support and training for women to continue this ministry of visiting the sick. Local congregations have Stephen Ministries. Hospitals, hospices, and some large retirement centers have chaplains.

As you prepare to visit those who are sick, you can draw on this Christian faith tradition. You join this community of saints. You share the living spirit of Christ.

Most people who are sick get well. While some people live into their 80s or 90s, some of them live longer, even with serious illnesses. Sometimes, when we go to see a friend who has a serious illnesses or who is dying, we don't know what to say. This book will give you some illustrations to help you know what to do.

DEFINING A SPIRITUAL CARE VISIT

A spiritual care visit doesn't appear to the casual observer to be much different from another kind of visit, yet the focus of a spiritual care visit is specific.

1. Spiritual care focuses on the patient. Its purpose is to add to, not take away from, the healing process. Spiritual care does not entertain the patient, tell stories, solve problems, give advice, or pass along medical information. Spiritual care listens, observes, values, and empowers the patient. What is happening that day for the visitor, good or bad, doesn't matter. Spiritual care pays attention to the patient, the patient's experience, and the present moment.

2. Spiritual care is sensitive to the feelings, emotional processes and spirit of the patient. It acknowledges the patient's feelings, pain, limitations, and realities. It does not offer solutions, teach or give advice. It does not declare "This is God's will" or "God wants to teach you a lesson." Instead it offers presence, love, encouragement, comfort and peace.

3. Spiritual care provides support and allows the patient to make a life transition. Illness may sweep a person out of his or her life pattern. Spiritual care represents God's love and care precisely when the patient feels lousy, is scared or is facing loss.

4. The difference between any other visit and a spiritual care visit is not precisely what you talk about, say or do, but that you do it in God's name as a representative of your church or faith community. For the patient you represent the face of God.

GETTING OFF TO A QUICK START

Confidentiality

As a spiritual caregiver, all medical information that you receive is confidential. You may know more than the patient or the patient's family. If so, you can't share this. You may know nothing because no one has told you about the patient's condition and medical staff persons are not permitted to tell you anything. Either way, you can make a helpful visit. You must be responsible not to share medical information with others. If a friend asks you about the condition of the patient you may say, "Sarah is critically ill. Please keep her in your prayers." "I saw Joe today. He's getting better." "Ron seems to be doing very well. He hopes to get back to work next week."

Before you greet the patient.

- Carry the address, phone number and room number with you.
- If you are going to someone's home, call first.
- Wash your hands or use antibiotic hand gel.
- Ask an attendant if there is any change in the patient's condition.
- Knock and ask permission to enter.
- Quickly look around the room for information.
- Who is present? What is their relationship to the patient?
- Is the patient on oxygen? (don't smoke)
- Is the patient eating? (you may give them a chance to eat)
- Is the patient awake? (you may give them a chance to sleep)

If the patient is three days past surgery and not on heavy medication for pain, check with the nurse or family. It may be fine to wake up the patient.

Is the patient on IVs? Plan for a short visit. You can get a feel for the length of a visit from the patient or family, but here are some suggestions.

  1-5 minutes for someone just out of surgery.

  5-10 minutes for someone awake and in pain.

  10-15 minutes average.

  up to 30 minutes if the patient is doing well and wants to talk.

Plan to listen. If you are talking, you are not listening. If you do not listen, you cannot provide spiritual care.

Getting started.

Greet the patient.

Call the patient by name and introduce yourself. This is helpful to people who are not used to seeing you here. It aids recall of your name and identifies your purpose.

  "Hi, Myrna. This is Jean, from Trinity Church.

    I promised to come see you."

Do

- Ask, "Are you in pain?"
- Ask about what hurts.
- Follow the patient's lead in the conversation.
- Follow the patient's feelings—anxiety, concerns, fears, interests, joys, celebrations. Paraphrase and clarify.
- Expect patients to do as much as they can for themselves.
- Help the patient reach something if it is out of range. "Would you like me to reach this for you?"
- Adjust a blanket if the patient is too cold or too hot.

- Remember that there may be different points of view about the patient's care, even within one family.
- Extend spiritual care to others who are with the patient.
- Allow for silence and don't feel uncomfortable. The patient will lead you.
- Ask the patient if they want prayer and if so, for what.
- Know that reading from the Bible can be very meaningful for people. Some people have heard these words over many years.
- If the moment seems right, share a verse or two from scripture, not usually more than about six verses.
- Ask the patient, "How can I help you today?" When sick persons want prayer, ask them for their prayer requests.
- Assume that many people are more comfortable with conversation than with prayer and that even asking people if they want prayer can make them uncomfortable.
- Pray in a language that the patient will understand or ask for a translator.
- If the patient asks for prayer, invite others in the room to pray.
- Take the patient's hand if that seems appropriate.
- Know that even when patients cannot talk to you, they may be able to hear, even if they are in a coma, heavily sedated, or nearing death.
- Maintain good boundaries at all times. Sometimes patients are not appropriate with visitors or care takers. Let patients who are out of line know that they are.
- Report patient misbehavior.
- Ask for professional help if you get into a situation that you don't know how to handle.

Don't

- Assume that people want you to pray.
- Pray if the patient or the conversation doesn't present you with the opportunity.
- Give advice.
- Fix problems.
- Sit on the bed.
- Flirt.
- Cough without covering your mouth and nose with your shirt or elbow.
- Give water, drink or food to a patient before surgery.
- Bring food unless this was requested, approved and pre-arranged.
- Don't bring anything with salt to heart patients, candy or juice to diabetics, or carbohydrates to people on a low-carb diet, etc.

- Talk about the patient's personal problems if the room is not private or the patient is not comfortable with sharing.
- Give out medical information. Use hospital guidelines for privacy. Let the patient or family guide you so that you know precisely what can be shared and with whom.

When you leave
- Tell the patient that you are leaving, even if she/he has fallen asleep.
- You may touch the patient's hand.
- Say something encouraging.
- "I'm glad you are feeling better."
- "I'll keep you in my prayers."
- "You are precious. Don't ever forget that you are loved."
- "We all want you to feel better soon."
- "I'm glad that I could come."
- "I really appreciated this visit with you."
- Don't promise to come back on a particular day or at a specific time unless you have built this into your schedule as a priority and know that nothing, not even a crisis, work, or a last minute important phone call will keep you away. There are too many things that could come up to divert your plan. Say, "I look forward to coming back."
- Wash your hands.

PART II.

Show L.O.V.E

SPIRITUAL CARE SHOWS LOVE

A spiritual caregiver symbolizes a holy presence with the patients, family members and medical care staff. A spiritual caregiver helps make God present to others and helps them enlarge sacred spaces where healing can occur. Patients need emotional healing. Patients experience loss, grief, worry and fear as well as sickness, injury and pain. It's hard to do emotional work alone. It's even more difficult if you are sick. That's where you are present as a spiritual supporter.

Your framework for spiritual care for people dealing with illness and death comes from your faith. God is love. Where love is genuine, God is present. In this book, the word L.O.V.E. will represent our spiritual care.

L.O.V.E. stands for four ingredients in the work of spiritual care. 1) **Listen** actively and non-judgmentally. 2) **Observe** with detail situations and feelings, including your own. 3) **Value** and respect people. 4) **Engage** others. L.O.V.E. is a way of using the spiritual caregiver's presence, interacting with another person, to enlarge the emotional healing space.

LISTEN

A calm environment and focused, healthy caregivers are good for healing. If anyone is troubled or anxious, healing is more complicated. Listening is an important tool you can use to enhance a healing environment.

When you go to visit someone who is sick, you may end up having a spiritual care encounter with someone else—a family member, a caregiver, or anyone who may be present. If someone is anxious, fearful, burdened or lonely, your time is not being wasted because it is not being spent with the patient. Simply by listening, you become the avenue for someone to work through their anxiety or issue. The patient becomes calm. The caregivers breathe deeper. You help model God's peace. Listen so that patients and family members know they are not alone. Good listening is at the heart of spiritual care.

One evening a hospital patient asked for spiritual care. When I arrived, the patient said that she wanted prayer. She shared about her life, troubles, children, and other concerns. She mentioned that the next day she was to be tested for cancer. I listened for twenty minutes. She asked for prayer. I began with a word of scripture. "'God will raise you up on eagles' wings. You will run and not be weary. You will walk and not faint.'" (Ex. 19:4; Is. 40:31) Before I had finished the first line she burst into tears. She said, "I know that you have the Holy Spirit with you." She described how that was exactly what she needed to hear. These words from the Bible spoke to her heart. They brought memories and comfort far beyond my own words. They had healing power. We prayed together. I offered words after listening.

She felt heard, and somehow my presence represented the very presence of God. When I spoke a word of comfort, she heard God speaking to her. When we prayed, she felt God was hearing and supporting her.

In the midst of crisis, people want to know that they aren't alone. They want to be treated with courtesy and kindness. Partial listening is disrupted by inattention, remembering "this reminds me of...," re-living the feelings you have had before, or lack of focus. All this fails to effectively communicate love and caring. If you are talking, you are not listening.

Treating a patient with courtesy and kindness is complicated. One patient wants constant attention. Another wants to be left alone. The entire setting of being a patient upsets ordinary relationships such as who decides, and who does what. Many patients want to do for themselves and don't want someone else making decisions for them. Sometimes well intentioned caregivers tend physical needs in ways that add to the patient's stress. To illustrate, if someone sets a call button next to the broken hand that can't operate it, this may frustrate the patient. To show kindness, you need to be as fully aware of the patient as you can be. You probably will not know everything that is going on. The patient's behavior or thinking may be under the influence of drugs. To provide spiritual care you must listen, sense and discern, sometimes making practical judgments, but not moral ones.

Listening helps build connection. Our culture tells us that people get to know us when we share about ourselves, but in spiritual care, our listening helps people relate to us. You may be surprised to discover that when you are able to hear a person's deepest concerns, they feel like they know you, even if you have shared very little about yourself! We share more of ourselves, not when we share about ourselves, but when we demonstrate that we care. Visiting someone is not about completing a "to do" task on your checklist. It is about letting people experience God's love for them.

OBSERVE

An amazing amount of information is available to persons who observe closely. Take time to find out what is going on with people. Before you enter the room, see if you can locate anxiety. Let go of your own agenda. By being spiritually centered, bring a calming presence that invites people to draw upon God's help and comfort in this moment. Your empathy represents God's comfort and peace.

Be alert to what is unfair or uncomfortable. If you were in the patient's shoes, would you be satisfied with your care? As a spiritual caregiver you may not be able to solve problems, but if you observe a situation that is more distressing than healing, it is appropriate to ask questions of a supervisor. Observe where there is anxiety.

Ben was dying. His wife and his best friend were at his bedside. I came to give comfort. Flowers by the bed, photos on the table, and stuffed animals given by the grandchildren showed me that he was deeply loved and cared for by his family and friends. Right then it didn't matter if the TV was on or off. No one was paying attention to the show. Ben had come to his last hours or moments and was slipping out of consciousness into that space between life and death. Cathleen was focused entirely on her husband, stroking his forehead and swabbing his lips with water.

Occasionally she spoke to him. "I love you dear. Are you too hot? I'm going to place this cool cloth on your forehead." Instead of taking time for her grief, she was caring for Ben. I made a mental note that Cathleen would prefer to be strong now and grieve later. Fred was across the room from Ben and Cathleen. He stood quietly, then walked up and down, turning away while silent tears ran down his cheeks.

If you were the spiritual caregiver entering this room, what would you do first?

1. Talk with Ben because he is the one who is dying.
2. Pray with Ben because you are grieving this loss of a friend and want God to help him.
3. Speak with Cathleen because you are her good friend.
4. Comfort Fred because he is anxious and crying.

Who needed spiritual care? Clearly, they all did. Ultimately, you might look for opportunities to provide spiritual care to each person one at a time. In this scenario, Ben was receiving care from Cathleen, and Cathleen was doing a superb job. Fred had the deepest need at that moment. The anxiety in the room was centered in Fred. Offering a presence and support for Fred reduced the level of anxiety in the room.

Fred shared with me that he had been diagnosed six months before with the same disease that was now claiming Ben's life. He was not only losing his best friend but he was watching what might happen at the end of his own life, and he was grieving his own death in advance. Fred needed time to be quiet in his grief and also time to tell his own story. I responded to his mood, being quietly supportive and listening when he spoke.

This was such a sacred time for Ben and Cathleen that it was appropriate to greet them and leave them alone to be in communication with each other. When she was ready, Cathleen would look around the room, but until then, a supportive visitor might be silently present, with permission touch her shoulder or squeeze her hand, and that would be enough. The spiritual caregiver might pray with sighs and prayers too deep for words, or silently pray for Cathleen and Ben and each person touched by Ben's dying.

Often family members are allies who help patients let go of worry. They may say, "It's all right. We're taking care of you. Just relax. We're right here beside you." This sense of coming home to loved ones and trusting them can help bring patients to a sense of peace. Ultimately, love is about trust. It's about putting one's life and well-being in the hands of others and in the hands of God.

VALUE

Good spiritual care treats patients and family members with respect. Showing respect means caring for others with integrity and truth. It means offering hope. Having observed closely what is happening for a patient, a spiritual care provider now helps a person explore his or her experience.

Maria was eating lunch when I arrived. She had come to the hospital with pneumonia but learned that her kidneys weren't working well. Her illness reminded her of her husband's hospitalization four years earlier. He had come for prostate cancer, but during surgery the doctors discovered that cancer had spread all through his body and into the spine. Maria's eyes grew moist as she remembered being married for 33 years. "He died. I'm all alone now." She described living at home and looking after various family members, but she dearly missed her husband. She was facing big changes, and probably would need dialysis. She had always been a strong, healthy person. Even though she was retired now, "I could do anything," she said. "I have cared for children and grandchildren. They are all raised. Now I feel so alone."

Spiritual care for this patient included listening and observing, but this patient also needed to be valued. Her self-worth had been closely tied to what she could do. She was anxious because she couldn't see what value she would have if she couldn't do anything.

Who you are is more than what you do. The Bible reminds us of this. You are a child of God. You are loved. Integrity is more than doing. It is being in relationship to others and to God. Sometimes it helps to remind patients of their true identity in God.

Maria was experiencing a crisis of grief and loss. Simultaneously she grieved the loss of her husband and the loss of her identity as a person who is capable. Spiritual care in this situation was about offering grace not always expressed in words. Through listening, presence, and understanding what the patient is going through, you offer grace. Grace was present in accepting the patient in this journey without judging, preaching, or explaining. A spiritual caregiver helps enlarge the patient's safe and sacred space.

Patients may need to hear the truth about their medical condition. Some families decide not to share this with the patient. One family decided that their beloved ailing eighty-six year old father was too frail to hear the news that he was dying. They instructed the doctors, nurses, hospital staff and chaplain not to mention anything about death or dying to the patient. They seemed oblivious to the fact that many people feel changes in their body and can sense when they are dying. These family members were grieving inside themselves, feeling and acting sad, but trying to hide all this from the patient. They felt that they had to leave the patient's room to cry or to make plans for their father's burial.[5] This didn't allow him to participate. Instead of showing respect for the patient, his feelings or desires, they treated him as an object of concern. Gently facing the truth about life and death actually shows respect for the patient.

Sometimes the shock of bad news is so great that a patient can't take it all in. A spiritual caregiver may help a confused patient by asking a medical caregiver to repeat information. Repetition helps people hear difficult news. Withholding truth gives mixed messages that prevent people from integrating what their body, heart, mind and feelings are telling them. Spiritual care is about helping persons be congruent and whole in what they are experiencing.

Sometimes people just don't know what will happen. The patient and family experience uncertainty. A spiritual caregiver can acknowledge that it is difficult to live with uncertainty. Christians trust that they are in God's hands, no matter what happens. Knowing that things are uncertain gives patients a chance to adjust, to make some choices about their care, to share what they need to say, and to do some very special things.

Emotional burdens stand in the way of coming to peace. Patients may be anxious about unfinished business or sins weighing on their hearts. They may have buried some secrets along the way. They may not pray regularly or be part of a faith community that helps them with the process of dying. Recounting unfinished things and secret burdens can help patients with this process of letting go. Many times there are broken relationships in families that have never been mended or maybe can't be mended.

Sometimes a patient has been a batterer or has cut off a relative for being gay. As a spiritual care visitor, you may listen to the story in private and must treat it with confidence. You may ask, "How do you feel about this now?" or "Do you feel as though you have forgiven yourself for what happened?" or "Have you made peace with this?" You may hear a confession and suggest that God has heard the patient. You may offer forgiveness in God's name. You may ask the patient if they want a visit from their pastor, priest, rabbi or spiritual care provider.

Authentic and healing spiritual care does not judge. As a visitor, sometimes you will hear things about which you have a strong opinion concerning right and wrong. Maybe someone has stolen, lied, cheated, or done wrong. Remember that this visit is not about you and your opinion. It is about the person who needs spiritual care. You may ask even-handed questions that help the person come up with his or her own answers.

One day I visited a very sick man who had multiple problems with heart and lung diseases and diabetes. His wife followed me out of the patient's room into the next room. "I want to speak with you for a minute," she said. "You heard my husband say that he doesn't believe in God. People from seven different faith groups have tried to convince him to believe in God, but he's proud that he has resisted them all. I'm worried about him."

I asked her, "Are you worried that he might die without believing in God?"

"Yes," she sighed.

Whose issue was it that the patient did not have a particular religious experience? It was the wife's concern. The patient was comfortable about not believing in God. The wife was anxious, and might continue to annoy the patient until she found peace. If peace represents God's presence, the patient felt it, but the wife needed it. A non-judging spiritual caregiver notices that it is the wife who needs the spiritual care.

I spent time alone with the wife. I asked if she thought the patient was at peace. She acknowledged that he was. I inquired whether she loved her husband, even if he didn't believe in God. She did. Did she believe that God's love was broad enough to care for her husband in the process of dying and after death, even if he didn't use the words she so longed to hear? When she affirmed this, she immediately became less anxious. Now she was free to truly be with her husband without this worrisome issue coming between them.

It can also be important to spend time alone with the patient. Even when caring, loving partners are helpful, persons who are ill may have concerns to address for their own spiritual care, but that they don't want to mention with the loved one present. If you are dealing with hovering family members you may be direct and ask for a few moments alone with the patient. You may also be indirect and say, "Listen. I'm going to be here for a while. Why don't you go grab a cup of coffee." Your time alone with the patient may be the moment when a sick husband is able to say, "I am worried about leaving her alone." Your ability to listen can help him express his fears and do his spiritual work.

ENGAGE

Spiritual care engages a healing response. Healing may include grieving the loss of a loved one or one's own approaching death. A patient or family member may begin to let go of what was and accept what is. They may confess their faults and weaknesses.

A dying woman told me, "I took care of everyone else in my family. I stayed up late at night. I got up early in the morning. I fed them, clothed them, cared for them, and saw that they had an education I never received, but I didn't take care of myself. I'm just burned out. Now I won't even live to see the birth of my next grandchild."

I replied, "I'm sorry it turned out that way. God knows you are precious, not for what you do, but for who you are. Maybe, after this close call, you are still here for a reason."

"Oh, I know I am," the woman continued. "My son just got out of prison last month. His employer and his wife have taken him back. He stopped drinking and is making a new start. He tells me that he couldn't have done it without my unconditional love for him. I need to tell him that I will never stop loving him, even if I die."

People who engage are on a good path. People who engage live thankfully in the present. It makes a difference whether people acknowledge and are thankful for blessings in their life. This separates patients who thrive emotionally from those who don't. Some are so eager to love and care for others that they radiate peace and bless everyone who comes to see them. If they have just had a close call with death they may say, "I guess God has something else for me to do."

Healing responses include experiences of grace, gratitude, creativity and calling. Patients and family go through a process of acknowledging illness or disability, grieving and recovering. Frequently sick people with a healthy attitude believe that blessings and goodness are unfolding in life; that God has something in mind for their life (a purpose); and that they are blessed and have love and creativity to share with others. They frequently talk about their blessings.

A patient once told me that he knew deep inside that he didn't ever need to worry. He must have come from a very wealthy family because he said, "My father owns all the land, pastures and the hills that you can see. If I ever need anything, I just ask my father and he gives it to me."

I thought, "Wouldn't it be nice if this privilege were available to me?" Then I realized that he was speaking of God, his heavenly Father, whose creation and spiritual wealth is there to be shared. It *is* for you and me. We *are* wealthy, and when we live aware of that abundance we experience abundant living.

Wholeness is about abundance. Spiritual gifts will never run out. They grow and multiply. Spiritual care gives people an opportunity to be filled emotionally by a spiritual fountain. By being the kind of spiritual presence that another person needs, the spiritual caregiver helps others access sacred guidance needed for life. God is the guide. Love is the deep channel.

PART III.

Spiritual Care to Fit the Situation

COMMON FACTORS IN SPIRITUAL CARE VISITS

What guides you to being an effective visitor is that without anyone speaking, you sense, intuit, know, and anticipate what is going on for the patient and focus on them. Regardless of the illness, patients often face uncertainty, loss of energy, pain, and loss of control (however temporary) over things like their appearance, performing ordinary tasks, walking, eating, and going to the bathroom. Some illnesses also raise the possibility of death. There are many scary situations including major surgery, major stroke, paralysis, heart attack, heart surgery, peritonitis, gangrene, amputation, cancer, pulmonary disorder, kidney failure, blocked intestines, brain tumor and meningitis.

Above and beyond medical problems and fear of death, virtually everyone who has a hospital stay has other compounding problems. The patient may or may not have insurance. Either way, he or she will have medical bills and unexpected expenses. Sometimes there is loss of work or income. Sometimes the car is wrecked. There may be a crime involved, along with a court case. Often a serious illness affects other family members in a big way. The spouse may spend nights in the hospital, or wear out caring for the partner or child. People in hospital may have pets needing care. Just when it is crucial for family members to pull together to support the patient, bad blood and painful family history surface again. Divorces, family cutoffs, addictions, crimes and secrets that are part of a family story are present.

As a visitor, you may never be told the precise medical condition of the person you are visiting. You may never see the junk that accumulates and becomes worries in the life of the patient. How can you be effective if you don't know what the problem is? You can. There are common human issues:

uncertainty, anxiety, loss of health, fear, loss of control. Spiritual care is essentially the same.

THE BASICS OF SPIRITUAL CARE

- Make an assessment of the patient's situation, level of pain, anxiety.
- Be present with the patient.
- Listen, listen, listen.
- Express care for the patient.

By your calm, caring presence, you show that the patient's worries are in God's hands and that when the patient is afraid and uncertain, God still understands, cares, loves and sustains.

"WHAT SHOULD I SAY AND DO?" QUIZ

For each situation, choose some appropriate things to say to a sick person.

Choice A

1. I'm really glad to see you!
2. How are you doing today?
3. Are you in pain?
4. Hello, Sue. This is Andrea. I heard that you are sick and I came to see you.

Okay, you are off to a good start if you used 4, 1, and 2 in that order, and then 3, if it is appropriate, as the conversation gets going. As a visitor, you aren't there to talk, but rather to give comfort. The length of your visit will depend on how sick the patient is. Quickly make an assessment. If the patient is not feeling very good, don't expect the patient to talk.

Choice B.

1. You look like you aren't feeling very well.
2. You look pale!
3. You have declined a lot since I saw you.
4. You look like you're feeling better than you did last week.

Sometimes patients look worse when you come for a second visit. There are many reasons for this. In general it is better not to remark on a patient's appearance. Answer 4 is okay if the patient looks a lot better, but the purpose of your visit has little to do with outward appearance. Spend your time instead looking at the patient's heart. Listen closely to the patient and observe details. How is the patient feeling inside? You might ask, "What's going on for you today?"

Choice C.

1. You mean so much to me that I wanted to come.
2. It's really hard for me to get over here to see you.
3. I've been thinking about you.
4. Everybody has been praying for you.

Responses 1, 3, and 4 all let the patient know that they are missed and that you care for them. Response 2 is about the visitor. No matter how much effort it takes for you to make this visit, telling the patient that you are doing this for them doesn't help your cause. Do not focus on your effort. Keep your attention on the patient's experience. If it takes you twice as long as usual to get there, or things are hectic at work or home, pray before you enter the room and center your attention in God and what is happening for the patient.

Choice D

1. Is there anything I can help you with while I'm here?
2. Can I make you a cup of tea or bring a glass of water?
3. Why don't you ask your daughter to come for a week?
4. Why are you feeling sorry for yourself?

If you are not in a hospital setting where nurses take care of the patient, and if the patient has limited ability to do things for herself/himself, you can ask if there is anything you can do to help, including bringing tea or water, however, never give food or drink to someone who may need surgery in the next eight to twelve hours.

Responses 3 and 4 are poor. Don't ask people "why" questions. If someone appears to be depressed, instead of asking, "Are you feeling depressed?" listen to see what is going on for them. Don't argue with the patient. The patient may be angry or grieving something. Allow silence. See what you can learn without asking. Wait to see what the patient is ready to share. After listening, you may want to check to see if the patient is self-aware. "How do you feel about this?" (Begin with a general question.) "Are you sad about this?" "Are you worried?" "Are you angry about this?"

Choice E

You and the patient have some mutual friends.

1. Kaysha and Ruth asked me to bring you their greetings.
2. Kaysha and Ruth think that you are depressed.
3. Kaysha and Ruth told me that tomorrow is the anniversary of your husband's death.
4. Kaysha and Ruth suggested that we bring Bingo over here tomorrow.

It is okay to bring greetings. It is gossip to pass along opinion, as in response 2. Response 3 is an important topic of conversation related to spiritual care. If the patient has not mentioned her husband's death, you might bring up the topic yourself. "Didn't your husband passed away two years ago just about this time?" The patient will give you the next lead. Carefully think through what might be an appropriate way to remember her husband's death. Flowers or a card might be suitable. As for response 4, don't rely on friends to tell you the patient's condition. They might not be right. Make your own assessment about the patient's health.

Choice F
1. I know a good doctor who could help you.
2. You can get the best prices on prescriptions at Save Big Discount Drug.
3. It's very important to get lots of rest.
4. Don't worry about things right now. Take time to get well.

Each one of these conversation points offers advice. When you give advice, it takes away personal power from the patient who is already deprived of his or her normal amount of personal power because of illness. Do your best to put choices and responsibilities in the hands of the patient. Instead of response 1, paraphrase, "You sound as though you have concerns about your medical condition." Instead of response 2, comment, "Prescriptions can be expensive." Instead of response 3, excuse yourself to leave by saying, "I can't stay longer now." This way you are talking about your own decision to leave, not controlling what happens after you leave. Instead of response 4, empathize with the patient, "It must be frustrating to have all of these problems right now" or "This is your chance to rest," or "Would you like to pray about these things?"

If you do encounter a situation that raises questions of justice, quality of care, or a patient's inability to pay for treatment, you may want to seek counsel, without revealing the patient's name or identity, about how to deal with the situation.

Choice G
What is appropriate to say?
1. I lost my husband five years ago. I know how that feels.
2. I had a mastectomy. I know how hard it can be.
3. I had my hip replaced three years ago. It has been an incredible gift to be free of pain again.
4. That happened to my daughter, too. It was really hard for all of us.

When you visit sick people, you will find points of connection between their experience and your own life. At first examination, all of these responses are not appropriate. If you know the patient really well and have already spoken about these things in another setting, adding responses 1, 2, 3, and 4 will not be necessary. If you do not know the patient well, and they are sick, this is not a good time to talk about what you know from having gone through an experience similar to what the patient is going through. Save your stories for another time.

On the other hand, each of the statements above is very concise. This much information might be okay to share. Sharing shows that you are compassionate and empathize. The two sentences in each example open a door so that if the patient wants to ask more, she can. Move right along to focus on the patient's experience. Your presence is more important than anything you say.

FETAL DEMISE

Fetal demise is when a pregnancy ends with the death of a baby before full term, a still birth, or a birth where the baby may only live for a few hours. Spiritual care is very important—immediately!

Modern medical practices have made it possible to save the lives of many babies whose gestation age is approximately six months. With a premature birth, the baby may be cared for in a Neonatal Intensive Care Unit for two or three months. When a baby is born at between 22 and 26 weeks' gestation, life can be very uncertain for a month or more.

A premature baby may have additional medication complications, need heart surgery, or experience hearing loss. Because so much is done to help care for tiny premature babies, women today are not very aware of the possibility of miscarriage, yet incidents of miscarriage are increasing. Many parents assume that babies will be healthy. They do not expect a death. That's part of the reason that fetal demise is such a difficult time for the parents.

The parents are overcome with grief and loss. They may blame themselves. Simultaneously they may blame God. They may be very angry.

Many possible scenarios may greet the visitor. You may arrive to see the baby's mother, before or after the baby is born, having just received the news that the baby is dead. The father may or may not be her husband. You may find the baby's father, grandparents, aunts and uncles present or being called to come. You may find a multi-racial family or a bi-lingual family.

The nurse may need time with the patient to talk about hospital procedures or take care of the mother. The doctor may come to talk with the parents about what happened.

As a visitor, you may feel a bit uncertain about your role. Don't worry about this. Focus on the people, especially those who are most anxious. The most important part is that you are present. You can say, "I'm so sorry. This is a big loss."

You may want to hold the mother's hand or ask to give a hug to someone who is crying. Ask permission, verbally or non-verbally, before touching. Some people prefer not to touch or hug. Be present. Witness the feelings. Ask if the family had named the baby. The doctors may not know the gender of the baby, but the family may have a name anyway.

Words of comfort may be appropriate. "I don't know why this happened. What we do know is that God loves you and your family, and loves this little one who has died. God will care for you and comfort and support you in this hard time. God will care for your baby."

Some things should not be said. Do not say, "God must have had a reason for your baby to die." "This was part of God's plan for your life." "God wanted another little angel." "God must be punishing you." If the parents were on drugs or alcohol, if the mother smoked during the pregnancy or lived dangerously, this is not the time for conversation about any of these issues unless the mother brings them up. Then encourage her to process her concerns by saying, "Tell me about this." Don't judge. Let the patient do her own work of discerning.

You may want to ask if the family would like to have a prayer for their baby. Practices in hospitals often allow the staff to bring the baby to the mother and the family. They may take turns holding the infant and grieving. An appropriate time for a prayer is when the emotion calms down after the family has held and looked at the baby for a while. If the baby has been named, you may use this name, praying that God receive and care for this one whose life has been so brief and that God will wrap this tiny one in loving, protective arms. You may pray for the family members that God will comfort them in their sorrow, understand their broken dreams and offer blessings yet to unfold in their lives. The words may be simple.

Sometimes the parents will blame themselves for the baby's death. You may want to talk with them about this. If you know that they were blameless, or think that this death might have happened to any couple's child, say so. "Don't blame yourself for Jason's death." If you suspect that there was parental irresponsibility involved, say, "This is not a time to blame yourself. Stay with your feelings. It is so sad to lose a child. We can talk later if you like." It is typical for people to blame themselves even if their action had little or nothing to do with the death.

When parents do process their own liability in the case of a fetal demise, it may be helpful not to have the extended family present. This may be a criminal case which should be handled by experts.

DOMESTIC VIOLENCE

If domestic violence was involved, talk with the mother. "Did James hit you?" "How was it that you were thrown down the stairs?" "Was he shouting at you?" "Were you afraid?" This is one place where it is professionally appropriate to offer counsel to a woman. "You do not deserve to be hit. No one should be hit. Together we will grieve the baby, but we will also take care of you. You deserve to be safe. This is a crime that has been committed against you." If the woman is under the age of 18 you are legally required to report domestic violence. You may not know all the proper steps to be taken at this point, but if you are in a hospital setting, the person to contact is the patient's nurse or the social worker in the Labor and Delivery unit.

CHRONIC ILLNESS

Carefully standing and leaning against the back of a chair for support, Lisa gave her faith testimony to her congregation. It had been a year since she had been able to come to worship every week. This once physically fit, tall, attractive, even-tempered woman had gained weight from taking steroids. Then she lost weight and grew gaunt and thin. She summarized her life story as a young attorney, wife, mother, teacher, and now a person physically disabled by lupus. She recalled the ways God had awakened her commitment to be a person of faith, compassionate and generous.

Lisa described how the doctor's summary of her medical conditions had grown from three pages single-spaced, typed, to more than six pages describing her illnesses, surgeries, medications, and chronic conditions. Bluntly, she named errors by doctors for which she had paid the price, and told how losing her ability to function sexually had been hard on her marriage. Her frank sharing helped everyone understand what she had been going through.

At that point Lisa was disabled, struggling to do for herself at home, and raising a pre-adolescent daughter, while confined to a chair. Blind in one eye from lupus, held together with metal pins, artificial joints, and a colostomy bag, Lisa shared her faith. God, who had seen her through injury, loss and surgery, was her source of strength. There wasn't a dry eye that Sunday morning.

I enjoyed visiting Lisa in her home. It was hard for me and others in the congregation to watch her health decline and to see her become homebound. She loved to read history. I found myself enriched by my visits with her.

I would prepare with prayer as I stepped into the car to drive to her house. I would think about Lisa and members of her family before I arrived and open myself to the experience. Sometimes I carried a Bible. Lisa always asked for prayer. Sometimes I also took communion elements after Sunday's Holy Communion, because this meant a lot to Lisa. I would knock or ring the doorbell.

The rest would be in God's hands.

At that point my task was to follow the leads. I'd always ask Lisa how she was doing. Sometimes we talked about her dog or members of the family. When it was time to go, Lisa inevitably expressed deep appreciation for my visit, and I always came away feeling filled and renewed. I marvel at this miracle, that God gives back to the giver.

The spiritual caregiver has many feelings and is often deeply touched by their encounter with a patient. You may remember a similar situation in your own life. When you are with the patient is not a good time to follow your feelings because you can't be fully present with the patient if you do this. It is not healthy to project your feelings and experiences on the patient or the patient's family. Give yourself permission to visit your own feelings after your visit with the patient. You may want to journal about your feelings.

TEEN AGE ACCIDENT

Sixteen year old Celeste had been involved in a serious accident. Miraculously, she didn't die on impact. Her right leg was broken but the worst part was that only two-thirds of her flesh remained on her leg. Muscles and tendons were gone. She survived hours of grim surgery and the news that she would be in the hospital for a long time. Day after day she clung tenaciously to life, fighting to avoid infection, gangrene, and loss of her leg. Her mother stayed by her bed around the clock at first and then day after day. Her boyfriend barely left the room. Her brothers came to see her. Doctors and nurses hovered over this very special patient who had so much spunk and personality.

Three weeks into her hospital stay, after pulling through intense trauma that nearly claimed her life, and after making remarkable progress in her healing, she reached a point where an inner switch turned off and began to give up on living. Her healing stopped. Celeste turned her back to the hospital staff. Nurses changing her bandages and caring for her just couldn't get through this amazing new barrier. Her mother and boyfriend just weren't enough support to reach Celeste as she moved into withdrawal. The hospital staff called for spiritual care.

This was not my first time to visit with Celeste, so I knew this special incredible teenager. I entered the room surrounded by a lot of prayer feeling that only God had the resources to help Celeste.

Celeste and I had a good talk. Celeste filled in some of the gaps in her story. The accident happened late at night. Her father was gone. Her mother was inside the house and didn't know what was going on outside. It involved alcohol, drugs, a former boyfriend, a new date, best friends, a brother, a motorcycle, and just enough jealousy, innocence, immaturity, and mistakes to make a nearly fatal combination. Celeste had been reviewing that night in her mind. She had seen how quickly poor judgment could shatter the present and change the future. People who had been best friends couldn't speak with each other. The costs of her hospitalization might bankrupt her family. Celeste had a lot on her mind, and she told me about it.

Almost all people have a history that haunts and taunts them with regrets. Repentance, forgiveness and acceptance are the keys to moving on. Healing depends on the possibility of being able to let go. It was with tears, grief, and anger that Celeste figured out who were her real friends and supporters and what she really wanted for the next steps in her life. As she came to terms with what she had learned and what were her deepest values now, she experienced acceptance and the letting go that comes with the experience of forgiveness. This didn't come across in her words but showed up in a sense of peace that came over her. Her breathing let me know that she had finished the conversation.

That day I gave Celeste the gift of a photo of a beautiful glass angel with giant strong wings. The angel knelt on one knee and reached down as if to lift up and carry one who is weak. The photo had a caption, "¡Si, se puede!," the Spanish for "Yes, you can!" The next day everyone remarked about how much better Celeste was doing. Healing and health are not far away from forgiveness.

HEART PATIENT

Kazuko was fifty years old when she had her first encounter with heart problems. She was wearing a heart monitor packet and receiving oxygen in the hospital. She shared how much her church meant to her, but then she spoke about her health concerns. She experienced low energy and depression that negatively affected her quality of life. Although she said that she wished she had more patience, mostly she wanted to get to the root of her health problems so they could be fixed and she could get better.

When I went to visit, Kazuko described an earlier experience with her mother that had made her angry. After so many years, she was still angry. She was angry at God, too, for giving her things to do but no energy to do them.

As Kazuko poured out her story, she began to reflect. "I need to stop worrying about tomorrow, stop trying to fix tomorrow's problems today. This is what God wanted me to hear today! I haven't been paying attention to what God wants for me, but your visit has reminded me of what the Bible teaches."

A recurrent theme in spiritual healing is to pay attention to the present. Energy spent worrying about the past or the future cannot go toward healing now. Kazuko was caught up wanting to solve problems by taking action. Perhaps one major contributor to her health problems was that she failed to handle each emotion in the moment as it entered her life. This meant she was spending energy taking care of the past and the future because she had not taken care of the present.

Mostly my role was to listen and observe. There are plenty of ways to let people know that you are listening. You might nod, lift an eyebrow, reflect the patient's emotion, or add "Hmm," "Aha," "Sure," "Of course," or other facial expressions or words that encourage the sharing without judging the content. This kind of listening is called "blank access." Good spiritual care brings out the healing tools and resources that people have within themselves.

When a patient is thinking things through out loud you might ask, "Do you think so?" Such a question gives them pause just long enough to think about whether they want to reflect more on what they said or proceed with their direction.

CANCER

Janet's doctor found a tiny speck on the mammogram. "Why are you scaring me?" she wondered when she first heard the doctor set up an early appointment with the surgeon for a biopsy. The surgeon found a thick area in her breast studded with cancer cells and removed it, but the report showed cancer cells right up to the edge where the lump had been cut out. Did cancer cells exist on what remained? Janet was barely recovering from the pain of the lumpectomy when surgery was scheduled for a mastectomy. The surgery effectively removed all the cancer. Healing the breast had to come from underneath.

Janet had been through more than a physical transformation. At first she felt it was her fault for getting cancer. She had taken hormone replacement therapy, which increases cancer risk. One health issue had compounded with another and she blamed herself. Then there was the strange new look of her body in the mirror. She learned that over time, the breast area that was bony, right down to the ribs, filled in with some fat tissue. Some of her womanly figure would return. "It took me weeks before I could say, 'I have breast cancer,'" she told me. In time she accepted the changes. "I found out that losing a breast is not the end of the world."

The surgery was followed by chemo treatments every two weeks for 16 weeks. Chemo zaps energy. It knocks out the immune system, so that a patient on chemo is susceptible to catching other illnesses. A visitor needs to scrub and wear a face mask. Gradually Janet lost her hair as well as her energy while she was on chemo treatments. Fortunately someone had suggested that she cut her hair shorter as she prepared to deal with being bald for a while. That preparation gave her time to get used to having a changed appearance. It took nearly a year for Janet to regain her health.

Janet was articulate about her issues: fear of death, fear of treatments, privacy, a changing body image. Janet had to develop a new set of spiritual resources to accept and live with her changed circumstances. Although she was open about talking with me after her surgeries, she kept her fears to herself in the first month. When you, as a visitor, see a patient, you can't assume that the healthiest process is to expect the patient to open up and talk about everything. Let the patient lead you to the points that she/he is ready to share.

DYING

When death stretches out over time—days, weeks, or months—the dying one experiences many emotions. She or he passes through a classic set of steps, fairly predictable, that include anger, denial, bargaining, depression, and acceptance.[6] People are angry to learn that they have an incurable life-threatening situation. They try to deny and ignore the physical changes. They bargain with God, "You can't take me yet." Depression may take the joy out of eating or enjoying things that ordinarily would bring pleasure. In the end, acceptance of death allows a person to tell loved ones goodbye.

Hospice has a very helpful guide that describes end of life in terms of changes that occur. There are observable ways that people wrap up personal business, talk with family members, have conversations with people important to their life, give up control over possessions, and value specific kinds of attention or affection. Human metabolism slows down, eating patterns change, skin color, body temperature and breathing change. Some people move from full consciousness to intermittent awareness and on into a coma. An observer cannot tell what the patient hears. Since hearing is the last sense to go, what we say to a patient may be an important aspect of a visit.

When you visit a patient who does not respond to your touch or your voice, you can still offer ministry. This time it's going to be you talking, but do also listen to the patient. Start with listening. Recognize that this is a sacred space where a person is almost living in another world. Sit near the patient. Match your breathing to theirs. Touch the patient's hand. Here's a sample conversation.

"Millie, this is Joan Smith from River Valley Church. I came to see you today. I miss you. I have been praying for you. I know that you are sick, but I don't want you to worry about anything right now. I am here with your family. Your daughter, April, is here with your grandchildren. God is taking care of you. God will take care of us, too. We're all here to see you through this time. Everything is going to be okay here. We are going to miss you a lot, but we don't want you to be in any pain.

"Your friends from River Valley Church have been praying for you. I want to pray with you, too.

"*Dear God, thank you so much for Millie. Thank you for our dear friendship.*

God, please take special care of Millie. May she never forget how much we love her. Bless her with your comfort, love and peace in Jesus' name we pray. Amen."

After the prayer there will probably be a moment of silence. Millie may be breathing a slow, noisy breath, the sort where, if it takes too long for the next breath, you wonder if the previous breath was her last one. You continue to sit beside Millie, holding her hand, and breathe with her. Try to feel her heartbeat and see if you can let your heart beat with hers. If you have more words, they can be spoken, but you may only have sighs and silence to share with Millie. When it's time to go, tell her you are leaving and let her know who is in the room with her.

HIV/AIDS

Mark asked for a chance to take the girls out for hamburgers. We used to have so many fun times together at church—the Halloween party, Christmas caroling, the girls swinging on Mark's arms on the church steps, and pot-luck dinners at Wayne's house. All that happened before Mark got sick. Our congregation had older members, and when younger people started coming to church, they came because the congregation had decided to openly welcome all people regardless of sexual orientation. There was one Sunday morning when a gay man shared that he had received a written threat. We had a meeting about security and trained the ushers to monitor the church doors in case anyone came to attack the worshippers on Sunday morning. The news camera caught 80-year old Velma saying, "I just don't see what all the fuss is about. We welcome gay people because Jesus taught us to love everybody."

Since St. Paul opened its doors, younger people came, most of them between ages 25 and 50. Mark was great with the girls, which I really appreciated. They learned how important it was to stay home on Sunday if they had a cold, because coughing in church could give a cold to one of their friends with AIDS who had a weakened immune system.

Now we rang the doorbell. Mark looked like a gaunt, frail shadow of the former healthy young man we had known. He couldn't drive, so he asked if we would. He wanted to take the girls out to Burger King for a treat, even though he didn't have a dollar to blow. The HIV cocktail had taken all his money. We talked and laughed, but I noticed that Mark could eat only two bites that day.

We saw him a month later in bed. Hospice was taking care of him. He was losing his memory and could barely speak sentences that made sense. He knew he was dying, and he made peace with that. His parents did not come to see the spiritual qualities in this young son they had raised—a man with a generous spirit and strong faith in God that helped see him through to the end. We talked and prayed together. Two weeks later he was gone. We had a memorial service for Mark at the church.

HIV/AIDS is still with us. When persons are diagnosed with HIV, they have an opportunity to take a costly "cocktail" medicine that slows down the development of AIDS. Probably there is more sense of judgment, guilt and shame around HIV/AIDS than other diseases or illnesses so consequently there is more rejection. Almost every church member has a family member who knows someone who has HIV or AIDS. As a visitor, one of the most helpful ways to be present for someone with HIV/AIDS is not to judge. Stay in the present, listen, and be present for the patient as you would for anyone else.

DEMENTIA

Gloria was an 83 year old member of our congregation who came down with dementia, a slow deterioration of her mental ability to keep track of thoughts or memories. We were close friends and had shared about our lives weekly in Sunday school. When Gloria could no longer drive, her husband Ted, age 92, drove her to Sunday school. I could hear them coming because Ted was stone deaf and always came roaring down the street at twenty miles an hour with one foot on the accelerator and the other on the brake. Gloria and Ted wanted to live in their home until they died, but Gloria would forget that the tea kettle was boiling on the stove. I didn't know how Gloria could cook a meal without burning down the house. In her hallucinating she had been seeing dangerous strangers in their home. Their only daughter, Susan, looked in on them once a day. At last Gloria's condition worsened and she went to an extended care facility.

I had just learned about this transition. When I arrived at the extended care center I saw Gloria sitting in a wheelchair outside her room. She was located at a T-junction in the hallway where she could see people walking up and down hallways in three directions. I walked straight toward her, but did not expect that she would recognize me. A staff person was feeding her lemon pudding. My purpose in visiting was to bring her love and greetings from the congregation, see how she was doing, and pray with her. We had prayed together weekly for a long time. I greeted the staff member and then Gloria. Our conversation went something like this.

A1: Hello, Gloria! It's good to see you. I'm Alice, from your church.

G1: Hello. I'm so glad to see you.

A2: I see you are the official greeter today, just like you used to be at church.

G2: Un-huh. And I'm going to come to church.

(The staff person excused herself and left. I sat next to Gloria.)

A3: That would be nice. Would you like a bite of pudding?

G3: Sure.

A4: This is nice. You get a bedtime snack.

G4: That's enough, now. I'm full. (Gloria took my very cold hands in hers.) Your hands are cold.

A5: Your hands are warm. Hey, that feels good. You can warm my hands! How are you feeling?

G5: I don't know what they're doing to Susan (her daughter).

A6: I think Susan's all right. She's probably helping Ted (Gloria's husband).

G6: That was so nice the other day. (The congregation recently had a special day to honor Gloria. She was homebound but received some cake, flowers, a card, and a copy of the bulletin containing her personal story.)

A7: You're such a special person. We all love you and miss you at church.

G7: Yes. I don't know what's the matter with him (Ted).

A8: I think that Susan is looking after him. You miss him, don't you.

G8: Yes. I don't know what's the trouble.

A9: Susan is taking care of everything at home, and you are getting good care here. I'm thankful for all the people who are helping you and your family. I'd like to have a prayer with you.

G10: I'd like that.

A11: *God, we thank you for your love and care for Gloria. Thank you for the doctors and nurses who are taking care of her. Keep Ted and Susan safe and strong. Give Gloria the healing she needs and a good night's rest. We thank you for your love. Amen.*

Gloria, it's sure been nice to visit with you.

G11: I'm so glad you came.

A12: I am glad to see you. Remember, everyone misses you and is praying for you. I'm going now but I want to give you a hug first. *[I gave her a hug.]* Goodbye.

G12: Goodbye.

It was hard to track what Gloria seemed eager to share of her concerns about people and things that were happening because her sentences didn't make sense. Because she hallucinated, I could not tell if she was talking about real events and people or imagined ones. It doesn't work to "correct" the details with someone who has dementia. When I didn't understand, I simply wanted to pick up the sense of her feeling and acknowledge it. Because of our long standing friendship I felt comfortable with a ministry of touch—holding her hand or hugging her, as she had done with all her friends at church over many years.

DIABETES

Many people have diabetes, a condition in which the body has trouble keeping blood sugars within a normal range. Blood sugar levels too high or too low can be a problem, lead a person to lose their ability to be clear-headed, or cause a person to pass out or go into a coma. Every illness and surgery upsets the uptake of food in the body, so diabetes makes healing slower. Diabetes can affect vision and ability to walk. Blood circulation decreases to the feet and may lead to numbness, loss of feeling and control. Diabetics are at higher risk in surgery, for getting bed sores, and for having limbs amputated because infections do not heal.

Because what a person eats is so crucial to the blood sugar level that must be tested several times a day, medical people keep track of whether a diabetic person is "compliant" or "non-compliant" in their diet. A diabetic diet should be low in sugar, fat and carbohydrates. There is not much room for diabetics to "cheat" by eating desserts and other forbidden foods. A visitor can know that persons with diabetes must deal with this disease every day of their lives. They can't eat most of the food served at office parties, happy hours, potlucks, meetings or coffees. For them, a vegetable tray is a great alternative to cookies.

Without excellent control of their diet, people with diabetes become "frequent fliers" at the local hospital. A spiritual care visitor may be tempted to want to admonish a diabetic to be more compliant. This usually gets a visitor nowhere. What works is to stay in the present with the patient and leave the topic alone, or, if the patient shares some concern about the diabetes, it might be possible to ask, "Is your quality of life declining? Tell me about what is happening. Is there anything you can do? Are you willing and able to do that or not?"

SUDDEN DEATH

Sudden death comes in many forms. It may be caused by a car accident or plane crash. It may have roots in violence such as murder, domestic violence, suicide or war. Death may be related to risk-taking behavior. It may come seemingly from nowhere and, with illness, take someone's life in only two days.

When death is sudden, the universal question of those who grieve is "Why?" "Why did this happen?" "Why did this happen to me?" "Why did this have to happen now?" Almost concurrently the bereaved person looks for a place to attach blame—blame God, him/herself, the church, the victim, the driver, the police officer, the President, the brother, the alcohol, the depression.

You, the visitor, may not be able to stop the "Why?" or the blame, but don't participate in it. Evil happens, accidents occur, and we don't necessarily know why. We have no ultimate explanation for why one person dies and another one lives. You may feel as though you have the grandstand seat for a reality TV drama and know where the blame belongs, but then again you may not be right. There may be pieces of the story you don't know or that no one will ever know. When someone dies suddenly and you go to comfort the survivors, hear them out. Being angry and blaming are normal stages of grieving. If it seems appropriate, you may remind them of that. Help them focus on their loss, and encourage people not to blame themselves but to deal with feelings of guilt later. Watch and be alert if a survivor of trauma or tragedy expresses suicidal thoughts.

When a loved one stops breathing, the family member experiences some predictable feelings. Here is one description of the emotional process that happens for the spouse.

Steve was at home when he stopped breathing and his heart stopped, too. His wife, Marilyn, called 911. Within five minutes the ambulance was there. The team started artificial resuscitation and CPR, put him in the ambulance, and rushed him to the hospital. At the hospital, a crew of ten people awaited his arrival in a trauma room. They gave him a sedative, ran a breathing tube down his throat, and turned on a machine to help him breathe. The doctor said, "All clear!" and a technician administered an electric shock to re-start his heart.

It happens every day in every city all over the country: Someone stops breathing and their heart stops. If the person is over 85 years of age, it is unlikely that the individual will survive the CPR, assisted breathing, and electric shock. The loved one has now died. If Steve were young and if his heart and health were strong, he might be revived. It might take a week or more to know if he is really out of the woods.

A person may be alive one moment and dead the next. It is a shock to see this happen to a member of your family.

While Steve is in the trauma room, Marilyn is sitting in the family room outside the emergency room, not able to be in the room while they work on Steve. She may be sobbing or have no tears, and will have almost no clear thoughts—only numb feelings. She needs someone present with her—the hospital chaplain, her pastor, you, a friend, or family member to stay by her side. You take her hand and offer a word of prayer that God will give her strength while she waits, and help Steve and the doctors and nurses. She pulls out a small slip of paper from her purse and her cell phone and starts to call family members.

A nurse comes to talk with Marilyn. "Is he alive?" she pleads.

"We're working on Steve. The doctor is with him. The doctor will come talk with you, but right now he needs to do everything he can for Steve. Tell me, did he have a heart attack two years ago? And was that a small stroke he suffered last summer? Did he have diabetes? Was he on insulin? Are there any other medical conditions you can tell me about? Did he have high blood pressure?" The nurse is rehearsing the health history both to gather crucial information for the patient's treatment and to remind the wife that her husband's health has been declining for several years.

After about forty-five minutes, the doctor tells Marilyn, "We did everything we could for Steve. He didn't make it. I'm sorry to tell you that he died." Marilyn sobs. "I can't believe it!" she mumbles. "We were just sitting in the living room and he suddenly grabbed his chest and couldn't get his breath."

Marilyn needs to tell the story. She tells it to the children, to her sister, and her closest friend. Within an hour, several people come to the hospital to be with Marilyn. The hospital chaplain comes back to the room.

"Would you like to come see Steve?" Marilyn turns to her dearest friend for a hug and cries on her shoulder. She nods, "Yes." They enter the room. Steve doesn't look like he did two hours before. He has a tube in his mouth. His personality is gone. Only his body is there, but it tells Marilyn that he is truly dead. She cries and grieves, maybe stroking Steve's head or hand, talking with him and pouring out her love and her goodbyes. Maybe she has no words, only tears and the hushed presence of a loved one who rushed to the hospital. Her friend holds her while she talks to Steve.

"Marilyn, would you like to have prayer together? *Dear God, we don't know why this happened, but we're really going to miss Steve. We ask you to receive him and take good care of him. We are thankful that he is free of pain and able to be at peace in your care. Wrap your ever-loving arms around Marilyn and hold her tight. Be her comfort and her peace. Bring her loved ones to her quickly and safely. Comfort Marilyn and her family and all of their friends and loved ones in this time of loss. Give them the strength they need in this hour and bring them close so that they can comfort one another. Amen.*"

When Marilyn kisses Steve goodbye and leaves the room, she starts to think about what is next. A member of the hospital staff may ask her if she would like to keep Steve's memory alive by making an anatomical donation that could give sight or healing to others who are sick. Marilyn may ask about what happens next, and call to choose a mortuary. She has made the first huge transition, but she'll need people to help when she can't think clearly or when she is emotionally unraveled over the next week or more.

Remember all the things you have learned about visiting. Listen. Ask Marilyn what she needs. She probably won't be hungry, but might accept a beverage. Offer to spend some time with her. If you are present, she may tell you stories about Steve (telling stories helps her to heal) or just be grateful not to be alone in their home.

CATASTROPHE

Our environment is handing out extraordinarily powerful catastrophic events including floods, freezes, heat, fires, hurricanes, tornados, and earthquakes. Add to these war, terrorist events, mass shootings, piracy and human trafficking. In your lifetime, you may be on the scene and want to help when death, destruction and trauma are all around. Neither you, nor the people around you, are equipped to fix the problems and make these situations "right."

One night I was paged at about 1 a.m. to come to the hospital to deal with the arrival of twelve people who had been involved in a van rollover accident. Ambulances were bringing in patients on stretchers. Accident victims were everywhere. When not enough rooms were available, patients on beds lined the hallways. One little six year old boy was crying and calling out in Spanish.

A nurse came by and said, "Mi hijo..., my son...." In very gentle, comforting words such as his mother and grandmother would have spoken, she calmed him and began to allay his fears. Later, when the nursing staff found that his nearest surviving relative was an aunt, they broke the usual rules and placed the boy in the same hospital room with her for their mutual recovery.

In times of catastrophe, fear and anguish can be addressed with spiritual care. Accurate, careful listening is important. Respond with understanding, paraphrasing, nodding, and non-judgmental words and sounds such as "Uh-huh, sure, I understand." Depending on the situation, you may be able to help by listening at some length. The victim may want help to contact relatives or friends.

Trauma is complex. Sometimes traumatized people aren't able to think clearly and need guidance to take rational steps that can reduce the possibility further injury or damage, such as stepping off of a busy roadway after an accident. People need to know that someone cares about them. After a catastrophic event, people may need a time of gathering for prayer and remembering to be able to move on in life. Typically, the distresses of trauma diminish and return like waves washing on an ocean beach.

Caregivers who help in times of catastrophe and trauma also share some of the trauma and need to learn how to release the weight of the traumatic experience. This compassion fatigue looks and feels like post traumatic stress syndrome. It is important for caregivers to take personal care of themselves. Hopefully, additional learning about trauma can be part of your preparation to provide good spiritual care.

CONCLUSION

Remember the four tasks of spiritual caregivers: listen, observe, value, and engage. To help you with these guidelines, this book provides resources and additional nuggets of information that can keep you focused on providing top quality spiritual care. You will find guidance for many situations; liturgies for dedications, baptisms, and Holy Communion; helpful words of comfort from the Bible and sample prayers. Additional books and resources are listed if you wish to dig deeper.

PART IV.

Resources

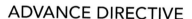

ADVANCE DIRECTIVE

Every adult should have a medical advance directive to guide doctors and families in the event that something happens to take away a person's ability to make his or her own decisions about medical care. Advance Directive forms can be obtained from hospitals and hospice organizations. One excellent model available in 35 states is called "Five Wishes." It guides family conversations about how to make crucial medical and health care decisions. As a spiritual caregiver you can offer forms for a medical directive to the patient or family. You may want to consult your local hospital, hospice, church or public library to see what is available.

PATIENT ADVOCACY

- If you have doubts that the patient is receiving the medical care that he or she needs in a hospital or nursing home, speak to the nurse assigned to the patient, not to the technical assistant or aide. If this doesn't work, speak to the supervisor of nurses in that unit. If there has been gross neglect, ask for the patient advocate.
- If the patient tells you about domestic violence or shows signs of being abused, share your concern with the patient. You may tell them that they deserve to be protected and that you will help them be safe. Stay with them while they call the domestic violence hotline. In a hospital, domestic violence should be reported to a case worker.
- If the patient does not have housing, care, assisted living, rehabilitation or a place to go when he or she is discharged from the hospital, speak with the case worker. If the patient is living at home and needs these

kinds of help, call the County Health Department for information about services in your area. With variations from place to place, Planned Parenthood or a YWCA may have resources.

PRE-SURGERY

- Check with the patient and arrange to come for a pre-surgery visit the night before surgery or 1 ½ hours before the surgery. The patient will be taken to surgery one hour before the surgery. Listen for the patient's concerns and concerns of family members. Be a non-anxious presence. If you are worried, too, take time for prayer and calm your own fears before you spend time with the patient. Put your trust in God to give you words of comfort for the patient, and offer prayer for successful surgery.
- You may want to wait in the family waiting area during the surgery to provide presence and support to the family during the anxious hours of waiting. This room is where the family will receive news about the surgery—whether it is longer than anticipated, whether there are complications, whether there are additional decisions to be made, and whether the surgery appears to be successful. The story isn't over immediately. People continue to wait. Your presence can be calming and supportive.

POST-SURGERY

- The patient will be in recovery for awhile. Later he or she will be moved to another unit. More complicated procedures are followed by a stay in the Intensive Care Unit, or ICU, before being released to a post-surgery floor.
- Provide a supportive presence.

HOME CARE

- Call ahead. There are times when a patient will not be able to visit due to how they are feeling or the procedures needed for their care. You may find your visit interrupted by their need for care.
- When you visit a patient in a home you are likely to visit with other family members as well. Be sure to introduce yourself again and state the purpose of your visit. You may want to include them in your visit. You may also want to ask for some one-on-one time alone with the patient.
- Sometimes home care patients don't like the care that they get. They may quarrel with their spouse or the care provider. This is not your problem. If the situation simply cannot be resolved by the quarreling parties, check to see if there is a third party person that they would both agree to use to help find resolution.

HOSPICE

A hospital, care center or home-based program for pain management and comfort care.

- Hospice is an amazing program because most of its services are provided free to patients who participate. The costs are covered in other ways by various Medicare, companies, donations and volunteer efforts.
- Hospice provides comfort care and pain management for people who have long term pain.
- Hospice care may be provided in a home, nursing home, extended care facility or hospital.
- Each Hospice patient has a doctor, nurse, chaplain, and case worker, plus additional help as necessary.
- Hospice care helps make it possible for families to keep patients in their own homes when they are dying or sick.

EXTENDED CARE FACILITY

- Get the room number of the patient before you go. Privacy is protected and often you can't obtain the patient's location once you arrive at the facility.
- As needed, sign in at the front desk and sign out.
- You may pre-arrange your visit or drop in, but if you drop in you may not find the patient if she or he has left the room for therapy, to eat, play cards, watch a big-screen TV, or visit a friend.
- Knock at the door of the patient's room. Ask permission to enter.

RELIGIOUS, ETHNIC AND CULTURAL SENSITIVITY

- *Learn about the cultural traditions of the various cultures in your area.* Use the internet, the library, the university religious studies professor and ask people. Talk with leaders from other groups about Native American tribal practices, African-American customs, African, Arabian, Indian, or Asian practices country by country. Learn about customs of Central Americans, South Americans, Pacific Islanders, Europeans, Mid-Easterners, Slavs, or Russians.
- *Ask the patient how he or she would like to be treated.* Are there special foods, drinks, or items for worship that would be helpful to their healing? If you do not know where to buy sweet grass, for example, ask the patient or a member of the family.
- Cultures have various forms of leadership in the family when a member is sick or dies. You can learn a lot by observing. Who do people go to for which kinds of decisions? Some families look to a man and others

to a woman. Some look to a daughter or son. *Don't do something simply because you see that it needs to be done. Ask first about what is appropriate.*

- *Ask permission before you pray.* A spiritual caregiver cannot assume the prayer is always needed. Prayer can be a pitfall! Many people are not comfortable with prayer. The family may have a mix of religious traditions represented. Catholics may want a priest. Protestants may dislike Catholic traditions. Jews may be offended if you pray in Jesus' name. Atheists may not want prayer. A relative may be a pastor. Include as many people as possible. If the patient requests prayer, ask what the patient wants to pray for. If other people present request prayer, first ask them to share their concerns. You may end up praying without ever naming God or Jesus. God is bigger than our traditions.

ASSESSING SPIRITUAL CARE NEEDS

- Good spiritual care transcends religious preferences and should be available to all persons. An excellent resource is the George Washington Institute for Spirituality and Health (GWISH) in Washington, D.C., whose director, Dr. Christina Puchalski, has developed an assessment tool for doctors and spiritual caregivers. Using neutral questions, patients are encouraged to name and ask for what they need. Questions ask patients to identify their faith or beliefs, what is important and influences them, their community of support, and how they want their needs to be addressed. This "FICA" assessment tool is available online at www.hpsm. org/documents/providers/FICAReferences.pdf and at www.gwish.org.

ORGAN AND TISSUE DONATION

- Organ and tissue donation gives life and health to others who have no other way of recovering. One relatively healthy donor's body may help as many as fifty to seventy other people. A living donor may decide to give a kidney or blood. A healthy person may decide that, when they die, they want to give life to others. Most donations do not interfere with the family process of grieving the loss of a loved one or interfere with funeral arrangements.

- *The most common donations are eyes, skin, bone and connective tissue.* An eye donation utilizes the clear lens from donors. Skin, connective tissue, and even organ donation is done unobtrusively with reconstruction. Even if a family wants to embalm their loved one and have a viewing, it is *unlikely that viewers will see any difference* between a donor and a loved one who is not a donor. It is important for donors to let their family members know their wishes. A visitor should encourage a sick person who wants to make an anatomical donation to speak with their family about this desire or intent if they have not done so.

- The simplest way to *plan in advance to donate* is to sign up with a donor registry in your state. Contact your Motor Vehicle Department or the Health Department for a registration form. Practices vary from state to state. Check the internet for other options.
- Here is what The United Methodist Church says about donation:

Organ Transplantation and Donation—We believe that organ transplantation and organ donation are acts of charity, *agape* love, and self-sacrifice. We recognize the life-giving benefits of organ and other tissue donation and encourage all people of faith to become organ and tissue donors as a part of their love and ministry to others in need.[7]

FAVORITE WORDS OF COMFORT FROM THE BIBLE

Psalm 23	The Lord is my shepherd.
Psalm 71:9, 17-21	You made me suffer a lot, but you will bring me back
Psalm 86	Please listen, Lord, and answer my prayer!
Psalm 121	I look to the hills! Where will I find help?
Matthew 6:25-34	Do not worry about your life.
Matthew 7:7-8	Ask, and you will receive.
John 3:16	God so loved the world that he gave his only Son….
Romans 5:1-5	Suffering produces endurance, character, hope.
Romans 8:35-39	Can anything separate us from the love of Christ?
I Corinthians 13:12-13	Now all we can see of God is like a cloudy picture….
Romans 5:1, 3-5a CEV	By faith we have been made acceptable to God. And now, because of our Lord Jesus Christ, we live at peace with God…. We…know that suffering helps us to endure, and endurance builds character, which gives us a hope that will never disappoint us.

PRAYERS

How to Pray

Ask permission before you pray out loud. Be genuine and authentic. Offer a few sentences in prayer, as appropriate, for the patient's healing and comfort, for guidance and care of doctors and nurses, for family and loved ones. Give thanks for God's blessings, love and care. Ask that God care for and watch over this loved one.

Using the Lord's Prayer

Many people are comforted by praying the Lord's Prayer. It can be prayed following any other prayer. Invite people to join you in praying out loud. Roman Catholics may pause before the last line or not include it. Presbyterians and UCCs will use "debts." Episcopalians and Methodists may use "trespasses." The variety is fine. People can adapt and feel included by sharing in this prayer.

Traditional Lord's Prayer

Our Father, who art in heaven,
hallowed be thy name.
Thy kingdom come,
thy will be done on earth as it is in heaven.
Give us this day our daily bread, And forgive us our /trespasses /debts
as we forgive /those who trespass against us /our debtors.
And lead us not into temptation,
but deliver us from evil.
/For thine is the kingdom, and the power and the glory
forever. Amen.[8]

Ecumenical Text, The Lord's Prayer

Our Father in heaven,
hallowed be your name,
your kingdom come,
your will be done, on earth as in heaven.
Give us today our daily bread.
Forgive us our sins
as we forgive those who sin against us.
Save us from the time of trial
and deliver us from evil.
For the kingdom, the power, and the glory are yours
now and for ever. Amen.[9]

A prayer with a mother and family who just lost their baby

(This may be one longer prayer, or a single portion may be used.)

Dear God, we have lost a loved one, already loved and known to us as part of this family before birth. This breaks our hearts and dreams. We wonder why this happened to our little one. We are sad and grieving. Help us not to blame ourselves or one another for things that were beyond our control. Forgive us for wanting to blame you.

God, please be loving and help us. Comfort **his/her** (mother, father, grandparents, brothers and sisters)_____ and all who feel this loss. Pour out your caring and understanding. Take care of us and bring healing.

God we ask you to wrap your arms around this little one so tiny and helpless. Make a place in your heavenly universe that is safe and loving. God, we ask you to provide the love and care for (*name*—or, *this child*)_____.

God, please use this time of grief and loss to bring us together for one another. Help us to be supportive and understanding, patient and loving. Thank you for your love that heals. Amen.

Prayer with a sick child

Dear God, we thank you for loving _____ and ask you to take care of **him/her** while **he/she** is sick. Thank you for the doctors and nurses and medicines. Help _____ to rest and not be afraid. Be like a best friend with **him/her** at all times. Help **him/her** be patient and listen for your inner voice. Thank you for the family that loves **him/her**. Help _____ get well. In Jesus name we pray. Amen.

A Prayer with a dying friend

Dear God, We thank you so much for _____ that we could have such a dear friendship. God, please take special care of _____. May **she** never forget how much we love **her**. Bless **her** with your comfort, love and peace. We pray in Jesus' name. Amen.

Prayer with the spouse/partner of one who just died

Dear God, we are grieving and we're really going to miss _____. We ask you to receive **him/her** and take good care of **him/her**. We are thankful that **he/she** is free of pain and able to be at peace in your care. Wrap your ever-loving arms around (the spouse who is mourning)____ and hold **him/her** tight. Be **his/her** comfort and **his/her** peace. Bring all **his/her** loved ones to **him/her** quickly and safely. Comfort **him/her** and **his/her** family and all of their friends and loved ones in this time of loss. Give them the strength they need in this hour and bring them close so that they can comfort one another. Amen.

Thanksgiving for Healing

God, we lift up our praise to you and thanks for your work in the life and healing of _____. We give thanks that your healing is made real and that prayers have been answered. We thank you for the skills and care of doctors and nurses. We thank you for the healing of body that also helps to heal our deepest fears and emotions. We thank you for all the prayers that have been prayed and answered. We pray in Jesus' name. Amen.

LITURGIES

ANOINTING THE SICK

The New Testament describes anointing of the sick as a ministry of healing. The key elements of anointing are laying on of hands, prayer, and using oil to make the sign of a cross. It is especially desirable to do this with others present, unless that is not possible, since the power of prayer multiplies when two or more are gathered together. You may wish to prepare for an anointing by obtaining a small vial of perfumed oil, although any oil may be used. Secure the agreement and consent of the patient and members of the family who may be present. Talk with them about the situation to discern the various kinds of healing, support and strength that are needed. You may invite people to offer prayers.

Typically hands may be laid on the sick person's head or shoulders, but if the healing is needed in a place that is appropriate to touch, hands may be laid on or near the place of illness. After the prayers (for the patient, for loved ones, for forgiveness, for patience, or whatever is appropriate) offer a blessing as the oil is used to make the sign of the cross on the patient's forehead. *The United Methodist Book of Worship* offers prayers for healing and wholeness, accompanied by anointing, that include this one: "May the power of God's indwelling presence heal you of all illnesses—that you may serve God with a loving heart. Amen."[10]

You may wish to conclude with The Lord's Prayer.

DEDICATION OF A CHILD WHO IS DYING OR WHO HAS DIED

Protestants believe that God's grace is present with the infant at all times. There is no threat of punishment, but rather an assurance of God's love for this infant. In this situation it is not necessary for the infant to repent from sin or for the parents to make promises on behalf of the child to teach the child about the love of God.

A minister or a lay person may arrange with the family to dedicate this little one to God. An appropriate time for a dedication is when emotion calms down after the family has held and looked at the baby for a while. The words are simple. You may start with a prayer for the baby and for the family members, and then conclude:

Dedication

(Full name) "_____, your parents and I dedicate you as a child marked by God's love and made in God's image, in the name of God, our Maker, Redeemer, and Comforter. Amen."

BAPTISM FOR A CHILD

Christian baptism is performed by a minister or priest who follows procedures and an order of worship provided by a denomination. Please consult your church officials or denomination concerning guidelines for baptism.

Introduction

We have gathered here today for a baptism. This special moment recognizes God's love at work in our lives. It welcomes this child and creates bonds between this child, *his/her* family and a community of faith. It encourages a nurturing relationship to guide this child. We begin with some questions for the *parents and/or sponsors.*

Representing the whole church, I ask,

Do you promise to model wholesome living for this child by rejecting all that is evil, turning away from sin, making amends for your mistakes, and using the strength that God gives you? Do you actively resist evil, injustice and oppression in all forms?

I do.

Do you confess Jesus Christ as your Savior, trust in his leading and grace, and promise to follow and serve him all your days, with the help of the Church that is open to people of all ages, nations and races?

I do.

Will you nurture *this child* in Christ's church so that, by your teaching and example, words and actions, *he/she* may be guided to accept God's grace for *his/herself* to profess *his/her* faith openly, and to lead a Christian life?

I will.

We continue with questions addressed those present who represent the congregation and we ask your response.

Do you, as the body of Christ and the Church, renew the vows made at your baptism? Do you reject evil, turn away from sin, and renew your commitment to follow Jesus?

We do.

Will you nurture one another in Christian faith and life, and now include *this person* now before you in your care? Will you surround *him/her* with a community of love and forgiveness?

We will.

(The pastor may give a short message about the meaning of the baptism of this child and the child's relationship to the family, the congregation, and God.)

Giving Thanks Over the Water

Gracious and loving God, your power and majesty have been displayed in creation and your incredible acts of salvation revealed through water. Your Spirit has separated water and land, filling both with life. You parted the waters of the Red Sea to deliver your people from oppression. You revealed yourself to Jesus when he was baptized by water and anointed with your Spirit. You have called disciples and followers of Jesus to share in the baptism of his death and resurrection. Your message of love invites people of all nations into relationship with God.

Bless this water with the gift of your Holy Spirit upon all those who receive it. Wash away *his/her* sin, clothe *him/her* in righteousness, and open the door to a life filled with justice, compassion, love, and fulfillment in God's love.

Baptism and Laying On of Hands (The candidate is baptized using all names except the last name.) "_____, I baptize you in the name of God the Father, Son, and Holy Spirit. Amen." Or use alternate biblical terms such as "Creator, Christ, and Holy Spirit."

May the Holy Spirit work within you, that being born through water and the Spirit, you may be a faithful disciple of Jesus Christ. Amen.

(Those present may offer signs of welcome to the child.)

COMMUNION

Providing the sacrament of Holy Communion to a person unable to attend congregational worship can be a meaningful and healing experience. While blessing and administering the sacrament is reserved for pastors, there are times when laypersons, directed by the pastor, may take the consecrated elements of bread and grape juice or wine to those who are sick or shut in. There are standard orders of worship for communion that may be used, such as those found in The United Methodist Book of Worship. *Typically a home, nursing home or hospital communion service is brief. The following prayers are provided as an example. "The Great Thanksgiving" is a prayer that recites God's saving acts and consecrates the communion elements.*

"Jesus, Touch Me"
A Brief Service of Holy Communion

Invitation

Jesus, our Healer, invites us to his table and into the presence of God's love. Draw near with faith, make your confession, and prepare to receive this sacrament.

Confession

O God, our God, who knows the secrets of our hearts and lives, we confess our shortcomings. We have hurt others. We have not believed in ourselves. We have neglected things that were important. We have followed the desires of our hearts instead of your call. We ask your forgiveness. Keep our hearts and minds focused on your peace and your people. God, speak your word that we may be healed.

Absolution

This is the good news, that God loves us and sent Jesus to us. In the name of Jesus Christ, you are forgiven!

Prayer

Just as Jesus touched the eyes of the blind man, helping him to see, touch the infirmities of our bodies and souls. Jesus, touch us with your healing power. Come, Lord Jesus, grant us rest and peace.

The Great Thanksgiving
(To be used by clergy or omitted by a lay person.)

O God, throughout history you have been our guardian, guide and healer.

When Haggar and Ishmael lay abandoned in the desert, hot and thirsty, you came to their aid.

When Saul's soul was tormented you sent David to soothe him with the music of a harp.

When Naaman came to Elisha, pleading for him to heal his master, you provided a healing touch.

When the people of Israel, held captive in a foreign land, longed for release, you gave them hope and comfort.

When a blind man asked Jesus for healing, Jesus touched him and opened his eyes.

When young men brought their crippled friend to Jesus, your forgiveness helped him to stand on his own.

When a woman who had bled for years touched the hem of Jesus' robe, Jesus' power healed her.

When Jesus died on the cross, you opened for us the door to resurrection and new life.

When you touch us with your love, we receive hope and healing.

You sent your Holy Spirit to lead and comfort us.

You have delivered us from bondage to sin and death.

You have made good on your promises in scripture.

On the night that Jesus was betrayed and led away to his death, he took bread, gave thanks to you, broke the bread, and gave it to his disciples saying: "Take, eat; this is my body which is given for you. Do this in remembrance of me."

After this Passover meal, he took the cup, gave thanks to you, gave it to his disciples, and said: "Take, eat; this is the cup of promise which is given for you. Do this in remembrance of me."

As we remember these acts of God, and God's love poured out for us in the life and death of Jesus, we humbly offer ourselves to God.

The Lord's Prayer

Our Father, who art in heaven,
hallowed be thy name.
Thy kingdom come,
thy will be done on earth as it is in heaven.
Give us this day our daily bread,
And forgive us our /trespasses /debts
as we forgive /those who trespass against us /our debtors.
And lead us not into temptation,
but deliver us from evil.
/For thine is the kingdom, and the power and the glory forever. Amen.[2]

Do This in Remembrance of Me

We remember that the night before he died, Jesus celebrated the Passover meal with his disciples. After dinner he took the bread and the cup and shared them.

Giving the Bread and Cup

The body of Christ given for you. Amen.
The cup of Christ's life-giving love poured out for you. Amen

A Prayer of Thanks

Lord Jesus, you have fed us with this sacrament. We thank you and give you praise.

The Blessing

Receive God's blessing. God has touched you with healing mercies and tender love. Keep your heart and mind in the knowledge and love of God. Receive the peace of God that passes all understanding. Go in peace. Amen.

HOSPICE RESOURCES

International Association for Hospice and Palliative Care
www.HospiceCare.com

National Hospice and Palliative Care Organization
www.nhpco.org

Hospice Net
www.hospicenet.org

Search the web for local hospice organizations.

BOOKS AND RESOURCES

Available from Cokesbury
800-672-1789 • www.cokesbury.com

A Hospital Handbook on Multiculturalism and Religion, Revised Edition: Practical Guidelines for Health Care Workers, by Neville A. Kirkwood. A succinct guide to the care of patients from a variety of faiths.

Bedside Manners: A Practical Guide for Visiting the Ill, by Katie Maxwell. Practical directions for offering care in hospitals, the homes of shut-ins, and nursing homes. Addresses care of children, caregivers, and patients who are dying.

Doing Girlfriend Theology: God-Talk with Young Women, by Dori Grinenko Baker. The author introduces a groundbreaking method of doing theology. Discern themes within the stories girls tell.

Forgiving Your Family: A Journey to Healing, by Kathleen Fischer. A psychotherapist identifies difficult points on the path to forgiveness in family relationships and offers guidance to work through them.

Health, Healing, and Wholeness: Engaging Congregation in Ministries of Health, by Mary Chase-Ziolek. Understanding congregational culture related to developing faith and health partnerships. Recognizing the potential of health ministries and promoting community health.

More Than a Parting Prayer: Lessons in Caregiving for the Dying, by William H. Griffith. Through poignant stories, learn lessons about the role of faith and God's will, grief and grieving families, faith-based denial, fear, different faiths, and dealing with personal loss.

Partners in Healing: The Ministry of Anointing, by Frank Ramirez. Provides a biblical and historical background for anointing, sample services, prayers and sermons to introduce this ministry to a congregation.

Pastoral Care to the Aged: A Handbook for Visitors, by Neville A. Kirkwood. An overview of the aging process, the challenges of dementia, and a look at unique emotional and spiritual needs of the elderly.

Pastoral Prayers for the Hospital Visit, by Sara Webb Phillips. A variety of prayers aid in speaking to the particular needs of hospital patients.

The Hospital Visitor's Handbook: The Do's and Don'ts of Hospital Visitation, by Neville A. Kirkwood. Strengthen the bonds of friendship while nurturing the patient's health, resource the patient's needs and moods, communicate effectively.

The Lay Pastoral Worker's Hospital Handbook: Tending the Spiritual Needs of Patients, by Neville A. Kirkwood. With Jesus as a theological model for lay workers, explore awareness of patient needs, ministering in times of crisis, and the place of prayer in the hospital visit.

Available from Upper Room Ministries
800-972-0433 • www.upperroom.org/bookstore

A Time to Mourn: Recovering from the Death of a Loved One, by Ron Del Bene with Mary and Herb Montgomery. A booklet with short meditations for mourners to help move through the "valley of the shadow," struggle with grief, and regain purpose and meaning for live without a loved one.

Abiding Hope: Encouragement in the Shadow of Death, by Ann Hagmann. Devotional readings based on Psalm 23 and reflections on positive ways faith sustains life in the valley of the shadow.

And Not One Bird Stopped Singing: Coping with Transition and Loss in Aging, by Doris Moreland. Death and tragedy are inevitable in our lives, yet our society encourages us to ignore our emotions during these crises. Coping honestly with our feelings of loss in death and diminishing body functions helps with inner healing.

Ashes Transformed: Healing from Trauma, by Tilda Norberg. Forty stories describe a wide range of faith responses to trauma on September 11, 2001. A helpful resource for anyone searching for God's healing touch and a resource for pastoral care.

Fire in the Soul, A prayer book for the later years, by Richard Lyon Morgan. A collection of refreshing and uplifting prayers that put into words the feelings and experiences of life transitions in the senior years.

In the Shadow of God's Wings: Grace in the Midst of Depression, by Susan Gregg-Schroeder. Discover new understanding of God's spiritual gifts that can come from depression.

Prayer and Our Bodies, by Flora Slosson Wuellner. Prayer both for and with your body and come to greater awareness of the interaction between body, mind, and spirit. Use prayer and guided meditations. The body can identify inner stresses and hurts.

When the World Breaks Your Heart by Gregory S. Clapper. Stories from the crash of United Airlines Flight 232 show how people found hope for living with tragedies that inevitably come to us all and came to see God's presence in the midst of these times.

Walking Through the Waters: Biblical Reflections for Families of Cancer Patients by Nancy Reensburger. Being attentive to one's spiritual life in the midst of illness can bring comfort and healing. Discover ways to sense God's presence during times of uncertainty. An introduction to several spiritual disciplines.

ENDNOTES

1. *The Book of Discipline of The United Methodist Church*, 2004 (Nashville, TN: The United Methodist Publishing House, 2004) Par. 316.1, 215.

2. Dr. Joan Guntzelman, "Your Wild and Precious Life," an address to the 2005 joint annual meeting of the Association of Professional Chaplains and the National Association of Catholic Chaplains, Albuquerque, NM, April 10, 2005.

3. Beth Cooper, "Touching Jesus," unpublished paper, December 6, 2005, p. 8. Matthew 18:20.

4. *The Book of Discipline of The United Methodist Church*, 2004 (Nashville, TN: The United Methodist Publishing House, 2004) Par. 301.1, 194.

5. Some patients want to participate in deciding whether they will be cremated or not, laid to rest near loved ones or have remains scattered. Other patients will ask the family to decide by saying something like, "It's up to you. It doesn't matter to me." The patient's wishes should be respected concerning what is discussed in his or her room.

6. Elisabeth Kübler-Ross, *On Death and Dying* (New York, NY: Scribner 1997. First published 1969).

7. *The Book of Discipline of The United Methodist Church*, 2004, (Nashville, TN: The United Methodist Publishing House, 2000) Par. 162, p. 112.

8. *The Book of Discipline of The United Methodist Church*, 2004, (Nashville, TN: The United Methodist Publishing House, 2000) Par. 316, p. 215.

9. *Ibid.*, 894.

10. *The United Methodist Hymnal* (Nashville, TN: The United Methodist Publishing House, 1989) 895.

BOOK ORDER FORM

Allow God to Wear Your Face
can be ordered directly from the publisher.

	Prices for shipping an order to one address	shipping and handling
1 COPY	$10.95	$4.00
2 – 4 COPIES	each $10.50	$8.00
5 – 9 COPIES	each $9.75	$11.00
10 – 19 COPIES	each $9.00	$15.00
20 – COPIES	each $8.00	TBA

Also available in ebook and ereader formats.

Also available, *Lifting Up Hope, Living Out Justice: Methodist Women and the Social Gospel.*

	Prices for shipping an order to one address	shipping and handling
1 COPY	~~$17.95~~ $15.95	$4.00
2 – 4 COPIES	each $10.00	$8.00
5 – 9 COPIES	each $9.00	$11.00
10 OR MORE	each $8.00	TBA

TO PAY BY CHECK, WRITE TO:
Frontrowliving Press
PO Box 19291
San Diego, CA 92159
619-955-0925

TO PAY BY CREDIT CARD:
email orders to frontrowliving@yahoo.com.